ANIMAL SCIENCE, ISSUES AND RESEARCH

FELINES

COMMON DISEASES, CLINICAL OUTCOMES AND DEVELOPMENTS IN VETERINARY HEALTHCARE

Animal Science, Issues and Research

Additional books in this series can be found on Nova's website under the Series tab.

Additional e-books in this series can be found on Nova's website under the e-book tab.

ANIMAL SCIENCE, ISSUES AND RESEARCH

FELINES

COMMON DISEASES, CLINICAL OUTCOMES AND DEVELOPMENTS IN VETERINARY HEALTHCARE

COLLEEN KEVINS
EDITOR

nova publishers
New York

Library of Congress Cataloging-in-Publication Data

Felines : common diseases, clinical outcomes, and developments in veterinary healthcare / editor, Colleen Kevins.
pages cm. -- (Animal science, issues and research)
Includes index.
ISBN 978-1-63463-550-9 (hardcover)
1. Cats--Diseases. 2. Felidae--Diseases. I. Kevins, Colleen.
SF985.F465 2015
636.8--dc23
2014043174

Published by Nova Science Publishers, Inc. † New York

CONTENTS

PREFACE

Cats, with a global population estimated at 600 million, are considered the most popular pets worldwide, and are adapted to all the environments and to different lifestyles. We can distinguish different types of cat populations, according to their living, which raise different concerns on respect to neutering or contraception. Feline Leukemia Virus (FeLV) was the first retrovirus isolated in domestic cats, and the infection is associated with a wide variety of clinical syndromes, including feline acquired immunodeficiency syndrome (AIDS or fAIDS). Inflammatory diseases of the oral cavity are common feline medical conditions and are associated with infectious agents such as Feline Immunodeficiency Virus (FIV), FeLV, herpesvirus (FHV-1) and calicivirus (FCV). The most common oral diseases in cats are gingivostomatitis, periodontal disease, tooth resorption and chronic periapical lesion by the canine tooth fracture. This book discusses the common diseases, clinical outcomes and developments in the veterinary healthcare of felines.

Chapter 1 - In this chapter the authors review the role of cortisol in the pathogenesis of chronic viral infections, such as feline immunodeficiency virus (FIV) and feline leukemia virus (FeLV). Cortisol is the main hormone involved in the "fight or flight" response, as it is released in response to stress. Its primary functions are to increase blood sugar through gluconeogenesis, aid the metabolism of fat, protein and carbohydrate, and decreases bone formation. Its effects on the immune system are also well known. It inhibits the production of interleukin (IL)-12, interferon (IFN)-γ, IFN-α and tumor-necrosis-factor (TNF)-α by antigen presenting cells and T helper (Th)1 cells, but upregulates IL-4, IL-10 and IL-13 by Th2 cells. This results in a shift towards a Th2 immune response rather that general immunosuppression.

All these effects have great importance in the pathogenesis of chronic viral infections, such as by herpes viruses or retroviral infections. Feline retroviruses are important pathogens of cats. Both feline immunodeficiency virus (FIV) and feline leukemia virus (FeLV) induce life-long lasting diseases in cats, which are characterized by the establishment of non-specific clinical signs (such as gingivitis, weight loss, cachexia, etc.) which might be a consequence of high cortisol levels. In fact, the authors have found that both FeLV-positive and FIV-positive cats have significantly increased cortisol plasma levels when compared to non-infected cats, but significantly lower than animals infected by both viruses. These high cortisol levels determine the shift of the immune response from Th1-type (adequate for fighting intracellular microorganisms) to Th2-type (associated with a poor prognosis).

As other steroids, cortisol is able to diffuse through the cell membrane into the cytoplasm, where it binds to glucocorticoid receptors (GR). Homodimer GR-cortisol complexes are translocated to the nucleus, where they bind specific DNA responsive elements (GRE) activating gene transcription. A second mechanism involves the binding of GR-cortisol to NF-κB or AP-1 to repress them from transactivating target genes. These two mechanisms are called transactivation and transrepression, respectively. They are responsible for the biological effects of cortisol, which depend also on the type of cell exposed to the steroid. For example, when GR-cortisol complexes cross the nuclear membrane of Th cells, they bind GRE which transactivate the IL-4, IL-10 or IL-13 genes and differentiate the lymphocyte into a Th2 cell.

Interestingly, retroviruses possess DNA sequences which act as GRE, i.e., they bind GR-cortisol complexes. They are located in the long terminal repeats (LTR), which are sequences which flank the proviral DNA integrated in cellular genome. LTR control viral transcription precisely by binding transcription factors, such as GR-cortisol. In other words, the virus is expressed in response to the cortisol levels in the cellular environment. Reduction in cortisolemia could be beneficial in these retroviral infections, but more studies are still needed to understand better the effects of cortisol in feline retrovirosis.

Chapter 2 - Though extensively used in the control of reproduction in domestic cats and in feral cat populations, medical contraception still raises concerns to the veterinary and the owners on respect to its safety and its efficiency. These concerns endorse, nowadays, the research in the development of new alternatives for effective, reversible and safe contraceptive methods for felids.

Hormonal contraceptives are intended for example, to master, in a reversible way, the reproductive cycle in genetically valuable cats, which presumes that they would be active for short periods of time and ought to safeguard the animal fertility.

However, hormonal contraceptives are also used worldwide to control the reproductive activity in either domestic or feral cats, for long-term treatments, because of a pretence short-term economical interest. Progestins are the most frequently used hormonal contraceptive in cats. They are quite easy to obtain in some areas of the globe and relatively cheap; they have diverse drug presentations, which allow its use independently of the veterinary assistance, and are effective in preventing pregnancy. Still some undesirable side effects on health are attributed to progestins when used in long-term schedules or in older animals.

In the past decade, several new approaches to manage cats' reproduction were proposed to avoid the use of progestins. Cats have a very distinctive reproductive function compared to dogs. Based on their particularities (reviewed also in this chapter), alternative hormonal methods were proposed mainly targeting to abolish the GnRH secretion, thereby interfering with FSH and LH pulsatility and the endocrine control of gonads. Two different routes can achieve inhibition of the GnRH secretion: controlling directly the GnRH secretion, by the administration of a potent GnRH agonist, for example, or indirectly by manipulating melatonin concentrations (since cats are seasonal breeders), thus mimetizing a lengthened non-reproductive season. Some of these approaches are considered devoid of adverse effects on the reproductive tissues. Nevertheless some secondary effects have been found in practice.

This work intended to provide an overview of the current alternative methods regarding the classical approach, for the control of the reproductive cycle in domestic cats, along with the presentation of the author's experience considering the feline oestrous cycle. Based on the author's common practice, the authors would like to discuss the treatment schedules, the risks found during its clinical application and the future perspectives of using these molecules in contraception. In the author's opinion this information can be of outmost interest to students, clinicians or colonies' technicians, breeders and even to common pet owners.

Chapter 3 - Feline Immunodeficiency Virus (FIV) is one of most common feline viral diseases, affecting wild and domestic cats worldwide. FIV belongs to the Retroviridae family, the most famous representative of which is Human Immunodeficiency Virus (HIV). The main mode of transmission is through bite wounds, but vertical transmission is also possible. Based on the mode of transmission, unneutered male outdoor cats are the highest-risk group. The infection is characterized by a long incubation period and a persistent infection, with development of acquired immune deficiency syndrome (AIDS), similar to HIV. In this stage the cat is susceptible to secondary and opportunistic infections. Infected cats may develop different clinical conditions, such as tumors and renal disease, but one of the most common manifestations is oral cavity disease. An FIV vaccine is available, but identification and isolation of infected cats is recommended as a preventive measure. FIV was isolated in 1986 in a colony of cats with opportunistic infections. Since then, relatively little research has been done on some aspects of the infection, like chronic or terminal stages of the disease, and mainly with respect to antiviral treatment.

The purpose of this chapter is to update, through literature review, some aspects of clinical, epidemiological, diagnostics and treatments of FIV infection in the domestic cat.

Chapter 4 - Inflammatory diseases of the oral cavity are common feline medical conditions and are associated with infectious agents such as Feline Immunodeficiency Virus (FIV), Feline Leukemia Virus (FeLV), herpesvirus (FHV-1) and calicivirus (FCV). The most common oral diseases in cats are gingivostomatitis, periodontal disease, tooth resorption and chronic periapical lesion by the canine tooth fracture. Feline gingivostomatitis is characterized by severe and chronic inflammation of gingiva and oral mucosa. The viral and immunological involvement in the pathogenesis of this disease has been increasingly recognized. There is a lower concentration of salivary Immunoglobulin A (IgA) in affected animals when compared with healthy cats. Thus, pain, anorexia, halitosis, weight loss and dehydration are common clinical manifestations in this important oral disease. To date there is no effective treatment. Because of its chronicity, the therapy should be individualized, aiming to minimize contact with oral bacterial antigens. Periodontal disease has no cure, only control. It presents as inflammation of the gums (gingivitis) and destruction of supporting tissues of the teeth (periodontitis), caused by the presence of biofilm. Treatment consists in removal of dental calculus and maintaining proper oral hygiene. Feline tooth resorption is an irreversible and extremely painful disease of unknown etiology. Clinical alterations are lesions of the enamel and / or cementum associated with severe gingivitis, usually on the tooth neck region. The most affected teeth are premolars and canines. Treatment involves dental extraction. It may be associated with periodontal disease. Teeth with pulp necrosis are a potent source of antigenic periapical destruction of parenchyma. Fractured canine tooth with pulp exposure requires a specific approach with endodontic therapy. The successful diagnosis and treatment of major oral diseases in cats depends on deep dental knowledge as well as the feline behavior.

Chapter 5 - Uveitis is the most common form of intraocular inflammation and a disease with potentially blinding sequels. Since the disease causes significant morbidity and the use of traditional forms of treatment is restricted by limited effectiveness and considerable side effects, uveitis remains a challenging field to veterinary ophthalmologists. Current understanding of the role of oxidative and nitrosative stress in ocular inflammatory diseases indicates that antioxidant and antinitridergic therapy may be important to optimize the uveitis treatment. Several lines of evidence strongly support that melatonin is a potent antioxidant molecule which is effective in scavenging free radicals that are generated in ocular tissues, and it inhibits the retinal nitridergic pathway. In view of the fact that melatonin lacks significant adverse collateral effects even at high doses, melatonin could potentially protect ocular tissues by effectively scavenging free radicals and excessive amounts of NO generated in the uveitic eye. This chapter summarizes recent investigations showing that melatonin prevents clinical, biochemical, ultrastructural and functional consequences of experimental uveitis, and which support the role of melatonin as a therapeutic strategy for uveitis treatment.

In: Felines
Editor: Colleen Kevins
ISBN: 978-1-63463-550-9

Chapter 1

THE ROLE OF CORTISOL IN FELINE RETROVIROSIS

Esperanza Gomez-Lucia*[1], *J. German Tejerizo*[1], *Juan Carlos Illera*[2], *Gema Silvan*[2], *Guadalupe Miró*[1], *Sonsoles Martín*[3] *and Ana Doménech*[1]

[1]Department of Animal Health,
Complutense University of Madrid, Spain
[2]Department of Animal Physiology,
Complutense University of Madrid, Spain
[3]Department of Animal Medicine and Surgery,
Veterinary Faculty, Complutense University of Madrid, Spain

ABSTRACT

In this chapter we review the role of cortisol in the pathogenesis of chronic viral infections, such as feline immunodeficiency virus (FIV) and feline leukemia virus (FeLV). Cortisol is the main hormone involved in the "fight or flight" response, as it is released in response to stress. Its primary functions are to increase blood sugar through gluconeogenesis, aid the metabolism of fat, protein and carbohydrate, and decreases bone formation. Its effects on the immune system are also well known. It inhibits the production of interleukin (IL)-12, interferon (IFN)-γ, IFN-α and tumor-necrosis-factor (TNF)-α by antigen presenting cells and T helper (Th)1 cells, but upregulates IL-4, IL-10 and IL-13 by Th2 cells.

This results in a shift towards a Th2 immune response rather that general immunosuppression.

All these effects have great importance in the pathogenesis of chronic viral infections, such as by herpes viruses or retroviral infections. Feline retroviruses are important pathogens of cats. Both feline immunodeficiency virus (FIV) and feline leukemia virus (FeLV) induce life-long lasting diseases in cats, which are characterized by the establishment of non-specific clinical signs (such as gingivitis, weight loss, cachexia, etc.) which might be a consequence of high cortisol levels. In fact, we have found that both FeLV-positive and FIV-positive cats have significantly increased cortisol plasma levels when compared to non-infected cats, but significantly lower than animals infected by both viruses. These high cortisol levels determine the shift of the immune response from Th1-type (adequate for fighting intracellular microorganisms) to Th2-type (associated with a poor prognosis).

As other steroids, cortisol is able to diffuse through the cell membrane into the cytoplasm, where it binds to glucocorticoid receptors (GR). Homodimer GR-cortisol complexes are translocated to the nucleus, where they bind specific DNA responsive elements (GRE) activating gene transcription. A second mechanism involves the binding of GR-cortisol to NF-κB or AP-1 to repress them from transactivating target genes. These two mechanisms are called transactivation and transrepression, respectively. They are responsible for the biological effects of cortisol, which depend also on the type of cell exposed to the steroid. For example, when GR-cortisol complexes cross the nuclear membrane of Th cells, they bind GRE which transactivate the IL-4, IL-10 or IL-13 genes and differentiate the lymphocyte into a Th2 cell.

Interestingly, retroviruses possess DNA sequences which act as GRE, i.e., they bind GR-cortisol complexes. They are located in the long terminal repeats (LTR), which are sequences which flank the proviral DNA integrated in cellular genome. LTR control viral transcription precisely by binding transcription factors, such as GR-cortisol. In other words, the virus is expressed in response to the cortisol levels in the cellular environment. Reduction in cortisolemia could be beneficial in these retroviral infections, but more studies are still needed to understand better the effects of cortisol in feline retrovirosis.

INTRODUCTION

Cortisol plays a relevant role in several infectious diseases. Cortisol is a steroid hormone, more specifically a glucocorticoid, produced by the cortex (from where the name is derived) of the adrenal gland in the zona fasciculate.

As the other steroid hormones, it derives from cholesterol. Cortisol is the main hormone involved in the "fight or flight" response, as it is released in response to stress. Its primary functions are to increase blood sugar through gluconeogenesis and glycogenolysis. It participates in the metabolism of lipids, proteins and carbohydrates. It also decreases bone formation, and suppresses the immune system. These functions are also shared by other glucocorticoids (GCs) such as cortisone or corticosterone and the synthetic GCs hydrocortisone and dexamethasone.

The synthesis of steroid hormones in the glands is controlled by the neuroendocrine axis formed by the hypothalamus and the pituitary gland, which secrete adreno-cortico-tropic hormone (ACTH) to regulate the hypothalamus-pituitary-adrenal gland (HPA) axis, or the hypothalamus-pituitary-gonadal (HPG) axis (Tejerizo et al., 2012). In the case of cortisol, the hypothalamus secretes corticotrophin-releasing hormone (CRH), which triggers cells in the neighboring anterior pituitary to secrete another hormone, ACTH. ACTH is carried through blood to the adrenal cortex where it increases the concentration of cholesterol in the inner mitochondrial membrane and stimulates the synthesis of cortisol and other glucocorticoids, mineralcorticoids and dehydroepiandrosterone (DHEA) (Figure 1). The HPA axis, as well as the HPG axis, is susceptible of being altered by different signals, either exogenous to the body or stemming from other systems, such as neurotransmitters or cytokines. In this way, the neurological, endocrine and immune systems are tightly interconnected (Figure 2). Each of the elements possesses its own molecular network of internal regulation, and the interaction with these signals may lead to its deregulation and the alteration of its functions (Gomez-Lucia et al., 2007).

Cortisol plays an important role in providing the body with a readily available energy source, glucose, from stored reserves by two different mechanisms: gluconeogenesis and glucogenolysis. In the fasting state, cortisol stimulates gluconeogenesis (formation of glucose, in the liver, from certain amino acids, glycerol, lactate, and/or propionate), inhibiting the synthesis of proteins. In other circumstances, cortisol promotes glycogenolysis, the breaking down of glycogen to glucose-1-phosphate and glucose, in liver and muscle tissue. Both mechanisms increase the amount of blood glucose available for fuel by the muscle, and allow the body to react to immediate danger or stress. However, prolonged cortisol secretion (which may be due to chronic stress) results in significant physiological changes.

Elevated levels of cortisol, if prolonged, can lead to proteolysis and muscle wasting. Its effects on lipid metabolism are controversial.

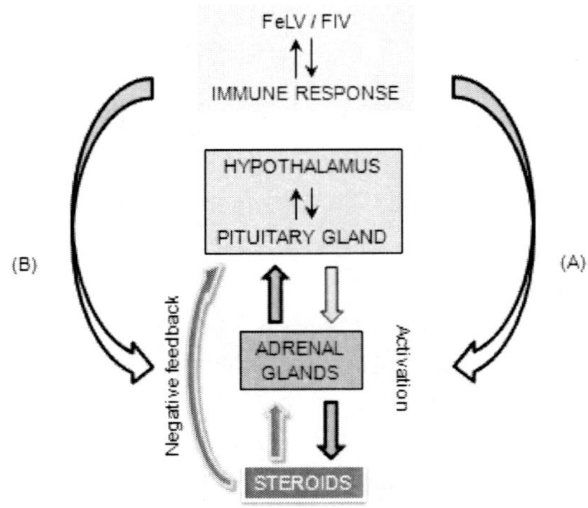

Figure 1. Possible interferences of FeLV and FIV with the HPA route. The relationship between the virus and the immune response of the cat could affect the activation routes (A), or the negative feedback circuits (B). Both events would affect the final concentration of hormones.

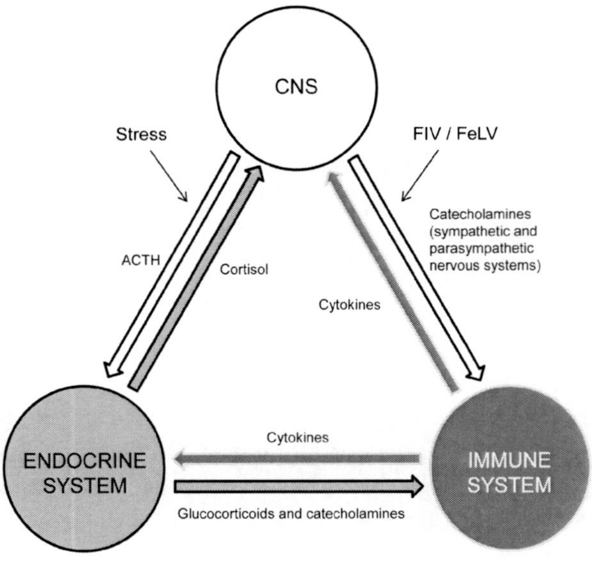

Figure 2. Network of three-directional communication between the immune, nervous and endocrine systems. Stress or an infection can activate and modify the proinflammatory cytokines balance, and stimulate bothe the hypothalamus-pituitary-adrenal axis (HPA), as well as the sympathetic-adrenal system. This induces the release of ACTH, glucocorticoids and catecholamines (adrenaline and noradrenaline) that affect the immune response.

Several studies have shown a lipolytic effect of cortisol; however, under some conditions, cortisol may somewhat suppress lipolysis (Bhathena, 2006; Mattsson and Olsson, 2007).

The effects of cortisol on the immune system are also well known. An important characteristic of cortisol and other GCs is their potent anti-inflammatory ability, repressing the migration of leukocytes and the activity of lymphocytes. GCs also reduce the secretion of histamine and stabilize lysosomal membranes, preventing their rupture and avoiding damage to healthy tissues (Yoffe, 1981).

Cortisol inhibits the production of interleukin (IL)-12, interferon (IFN)-γ, IFN-α and tumor-necrosis-factor (TNF) α by antigen presenting cells and T helper (Th)1 cells. On the other hand, it upregulates IL-4, IL-10 and IL-13 secretion by Th2 cells. This results in a shift towards a Th2 immune response rather that general immunosuppression. In addition, it prevents the proliferation of T-cells by rendering the IL-2 producer T-cells unresponsive to IL-1 and unable to produce the T-cell growth factor (TCGF) (Dimitrov et al., 2004). The activation of the stress system (and resulting increase in cortisol and Th2 shift) seen during an infection is believed to be a protective mechanism which prevents an over activation of the inflammatory response.

For all these reasons, GCs are used to treat inflammatory diseases resulting from over activity of the B-cell-mediated antibody response. Examples include inflammatory and rheumatoid diseases, as well as allergies, but also certain types of leukemia and lymphomas (Gomez-Lucia et al., 2007).

Feline Leukemia and Feline Immunodeficiency

Both feline immunodeficiency and feline leukemia have aspects in common: they are chronic and persistent infections affecting mainly lymphocytes and other cells of the immune system, and are characterized by a variety of signs that are clinically nonspecific. Besides, the excess of circulating immune complexes which develop in both infections could contribute to the immune mediated lesions and signs associated with the infection by any of these two viruses. The clinical signs are further confused by the possibility of animals infected by both viruses or double infected. In spite of these similarities, the pathogenic mechanisms of both viruses are quite different and not completely understood yet.

FIV usually is transmitted through bites and wounds produced by aggressions between cats. The infection progresses slowly through several stages during several months or even years, although there is no clear distinction between these stages in naturally infected cats, and in most animals it does not adversely affect the cats' life expectancy (Hartmann, 2012). After an initial replication in the regional lymph nodes and other lymphoid organs, a short initial viremia occurs in which the virus is spread throughout the body, infecting lymphocytes, monocytes and macrophages of the bone marrow, intestinal tract, lung, kidney and brain ("initial stage" or "acute phase"). A few weeks later, the cat develops a cellular and humoral immune response which, however, fails to completely eliminate the virus. This acute phase, which generally lasts four to six weeks but can persist up to one year, is characterized by transient or mild clinical signs, as hyperthermia, lethargy, generalized lymphadenopathy, stomatitis, diarrhea, depression, skin lesions, intraocular inflammation, variable neurologic signs, etc. (Domenech et al., 2012; Lawson and Hosie, 2001).

The infection progresses slowly to a chronic subclinical period, which corresponds to the "phase of clinical latency", with low levels of viral expression. This period can last from months to many years and even may be lifelong lasting in some animals. During this subclinical phase, the immune system weakens gradually, with a progressive decrease of $CD4^+$ T-cells (due to direct replication of the virus in these cells) which leads to lymphopenia and inversion of the CD4/CD8 ratio, along with a decrease in the functionality of infected lymphocytes. In most FIV-infected cats, there is a marked hypergammaglobulinemia, primarily due to the polyclonal stimulation of B-cells which give rise to an increase of IgG not specific to FIV (Miró et al., 2007). As infection progresses, mild clinical signs, such as relapsing fever, leucopenia, lymphadenopathy, anorexia, weight loss, etc. may develop. At the end of this stage, the clinical triad lymphadenopathy-gingivitis-hypergammaglobulinemia may be observed (Collado et al., 2012; Domenech et al., 2012; Gleich and Hartmann, 2009; Hartmann, 2011, 2012).

In some infected cats, often many years after infection and coinciding with very low values of CD4/CD8, plasma viremia increases, leading to a terminal phase, the so-called "feline acquired immunodeficiency syndrome" or FAIDS, due to its resemblance to human AIDS (Hartmann, 2011, 2012). During this stage with clinical signs the lymphocyte depletion is much more pronounced and opportunistic infections occur, against which the cat cannot develop an adequate immune response. Multiple chronic infections are observed, such as gingivo-stomatitis, respiratory diseases, pyodermas, or disorders of the nervous system, the kidneys, the eyes, etc. When the CD4/CD8 ratio decreases further, acquired immunodeficiency develops, and tumors, such as squamous cells carcinoma and lymphoma, neurologic and several immune-mediated clinical signs may be detected (uveitis, glomerulonephritis, cholangitis, etc.), although very few are due to direct viral action (Hartmann, 2011, 2012; Lawson and Hosie, 2001). Cats which suffer FAIDS die from a chronic syndrome of wasting, neurological disease, neoplasia or systemic opportunistic infections (Domenech et al., 2012; Dunham and Graham, 2008; Hartmann, 2011, 2012).

Saliva is the main source of infection for FeLV, as viremic cats with or without clinical signs shed constantly viral particles through it (Hartmann, 2011). For this reason, mutual grooming or sharing food or water bowls are risk factors for FeLV transmission. The animal usually gets infected by the oronasal route, and the virus replicates in the local oropharyngeal lymphoid tissue. The outcome of FeLV infection is very different in each cat, as it depends on factors related to both the virus (subgroup of FeLV, duration of exposure and infective viral load) and the host (age and immune status) (Dunham and Graham, 2008; Hartmann, 2011). Most cats develop an effective immune response, but in very few of them the virus is completely cleared from the body at a very early stage ("abortive infection") and animals never become viremic. After the initial replication, there is a transient viremia in which the virus infects lymphocytes and monocytes, and is spread to different tissues (spleen, thymus, salivary glands, lymph nodes) ("regressive infection"). However, in some cats viremia persists longer than three weeks and FeLV infects bone marrow stem cells, producing a massive replication of the virus and the development of persistent viremia (both of free virus and of infected cells), which gives rise to "persistent or progressive infection". In this phase, the virus infection cannot be completely eliminated because the provirus is present in the stem cells in the bone marrow. In addition, hematopoietic alterations (particularly cytopenias) are produced, caused by the suppression of the bone marrow as a result of the infection (Hartmann, 2011, 2012). An unknown percentage of cats develop a "latent infection", in which, although the bone marrow becomes infected, it does not release virus or infected cells. These animals remain apparently healthy until the provirus is reactivated by an immunosuppressor or treatment. Very young cats are more likely to develop a progressive infection, probably due to their immature immune system, while older cats tend to develop a regressive or abortive infection. Atypical infections in which the virus is located in organs, as the bladder, eyes or the mammary gland, partially hidden from an effective immune response, have been described in a very low number of animals.

The clinical signs in FeLV persistently infected cats are more specific than those observed in the course of FIV infection and the evolution is faster, and these cats usually die in 1-3 years from a disease related to FeLV infection, including neoplastic and/or non-neoplastic disease. FeLV is an oncogenic virus which may induce several types of neoplasias, of which lymphoma and lymphoblastic leukemia are the most prevalent. Besides that, myeloproliferative neoplasias, fibrosarcoma, osteochondroma and neuroblastoma have also been described in infected cats (Collado et al., 2012; Hartmann, 2011, 2012; Hofmann-Lehmann et al., 2007).

Non-neoplastic diseases include hematologic disorders, immune-suppression, immune-mediated diseases and other syndromes, as neuropathy and reproductive disorders. Anemia is frequently observed in viremic cats and could be predictive of imminent death. It may be non-regenerative (as a result of myelosuppression, myelodestruction, or myeloproliferative diseases) or hemolytic (immune-mediated or secondary to *Mycoplasma haemofelis* infection) (Hartmann, 2011; Hofmann-Lehmann et al., 2007). Lymphonenia and neutropenia are also common (Collado et al., 2012). Immunosuppression may be caused by different mechanisms and it is mainly associated with some variants of the virus. Certain immunosuppressive FeLV strains (FeLV-T), with a strong tropism for T-cells, have also been reported to induce an acquired immunodeficiency syndrome similar to the one produced by FIV (Hartmann, 2011). The immunosuppression predisposes animals to secondary infections, such as stomatitis, abscesses, pyothorax, dermatitis, feline infectious peritonitis, toxoplasmosis or cryptococcosis. Some immune-mediated alterations observed in FeLV positive cats are autoimmune glomerulonefritis, uveitis and neutrophilic polyarthritis (Hartmann, 2011; Hofmann-Lehmann et al., 2007). In regards to reproductive disorders, FeLV infection may also cause infertility and abortions, and newborn kittens are frequently lethargic. Nowadays, most of persistently infected cats show anemia, immunosuppresive or immune-mediated disorders instead of tumors (Hartmann, 2011).

Both retroviral infections in cats induce deep deregulation of the functions of the immune system, probably associated with changes in the cytokine pattern, especially described in FIV infections. Increased TNFα and altered levels of IFN-γ, IL-2, IL-4, IL-6 are observed in FeLV and FIV infected cats (Hartmann, 2011; Levy et al., 2004; Linenberger and Deng, 1999). Proinflammatory cytokines (IL-6, TNFα) may also contribute to illness. Increased IL-10/IL-12 ratio (due to an increase of IL-10) found in FIV infection is associated to the shift from type Th1 to response (which restrains disease progression) to type Th2 (which allows disease progression) during

FIV progression (Levy et al., 2004, 2004). The excessive production of the Th2 type cytokine IL-10 may also induce the production of glucocorticoids indirectly (via the release of cortisol releasing hormone, CRH, and/or ACTH) or directly by stimulating adrenal glucocorticoid biosynthesis, which could be also associated with the evolution of infection. As cortisol suppresses cell-mediated immunity and may stimulate humoral immunity, its increase could be detrimental in FIV infection.

CORTISOL IN FIV AND FELV INFECTIONS

In general, viral infections increase cortisol levels through activation of the HPA axis by cytokines (Silverman et al., 2005). Infections by FIV or FeLV are no exception to this. Diseases produced by these pathogens are also paradigmatic in the sense that they are chronic, long-lasting infections, which produce a continuous activation of the immune system. However, there are few studies which focus on hormonal alterations resulting from infection by feline retroviruses. Teng (1990) reported both increases and decreases in the plasma concentration of cortisol and ACTH in FeLV-infected cats, which depended on the stage of the disease. They were attributed to the absence of adrenal response to the pituitary orders.

In the case of FIV, to the best of our knowledge, these types of studies are non-existent. Recently, our research group has obtained the results shown below.

Cortisol levels were determined in the serum or plasma of cats naturally infected by FIV (9 female and 33 male cats), FeLV (26 female and 17 male cats), or FIV and FeLV-infected (6 female and 6 male cats), as well as non-infected (38 females and 35 male cats) using a competitive EIA technique (Tejerizo et al., 2012). Retroviral infection was diagnosed using Snap Combo (Idexx) and a double-nested PCR designed by our group (Arjona et al., 2007). Statistically significant differences in cortisol levels between infected and non-infected cats were observed. Cortisol levels in non-infected, FeLV-positive (FeLV+), FIV-positive (FIV+) and FeLV and FIV-positive (F-F) cats were an average of 53, 213, 217 and 662 ng/mL, respectively; *i.e.* 4x higher in cats infected by either FIV or FeLV and 12x in double-infected cats than in non-infected animals (Figure 3A). Generally, infected male cats had higher cortisol plasma concentrations than infected female cats (Figure 3B) (differences between males and females were statistically significant, $p<0.05$, in FeLV+ cats). FIV-infected cats with clinical signs had lower cortisol plasma concentration than FIV-infected cats without clinical signs, but differences were not statistically significant (Figure 3C). The highest cortisol concentrations (850-1290 ng/mL) were found in three FIV+ cats, but no pattern according to sex, age, or presence/absence of clinical signs could be established. The small range of variation of the concentration of plasma cortisol in each of the groups (non-infected, FeLV+, FIV+, F-F; Table 1) was surprising. This was regardless of the time of the day in which the blood samples were taken, the vaccination status, stress, being stray or home-kept, or any other circumstance which usually affects cortisol concentration.

Diurnal cycles of cortisol levels are found in several animal species. In species that exhibit such cycles, different timing of diurnal maxima and minima has been observed, not only in different species (Martin, P.A. and Crump, M.H., 2003) but also, in some cases, within the same species (Fulkerson and Tang, 1979; Mesbah and Brudieux, 1982; Simonetta et al., 1991; Stella et al., 2013). The variations are due to the information about the light/dark cycles, transmitted from the retina.

Though there are few data about cortisol levels in FIV-infected cats, cortisol concentrations have been analyzed in individuals infected with the closely related lentivirus HIV. Endocrine dysfunctions have also been observed in HIV-positive patients. It is known that in the case of HIV many of the clinical signs associated to the infection are similar to those derived from an excessive production of GCs. In general, with a few exceptions, data show a clear increase of cortisol and decrease of dehydro-epi-androsterone (DHEA) concentrations in all HIV-1 patients, regardless of the stage of the disease and the treatment administered (Abrams et al., 2007; Bons et al., 2013; Chittiprol et al., 2007, 2009; Christeff et al., 2000, 2002a; Clerici et al., 2000; Laudat et al., 1995; Schifitto et al., 2000). This phenomenon seems to be accompanied by high levels of estrogens (Christeff et al., 1992; Poretsky et al., 2009; Teichmann et al., 1998) and reduced levels of testosterone (Christeff et al., 1992; Laudat et al., 1995; Poretsky et al., 1995; Villette et al., 1990).

Cortisol / DHEA Ratio

DHEA is another steroid hormone, secreted by the adrenal cortex, the gonads and the brain, where it functions predominantly as a metabolic intermediate in the biosynthesis of androgen and estrogen sex steroids (Domenech et al., 2009).

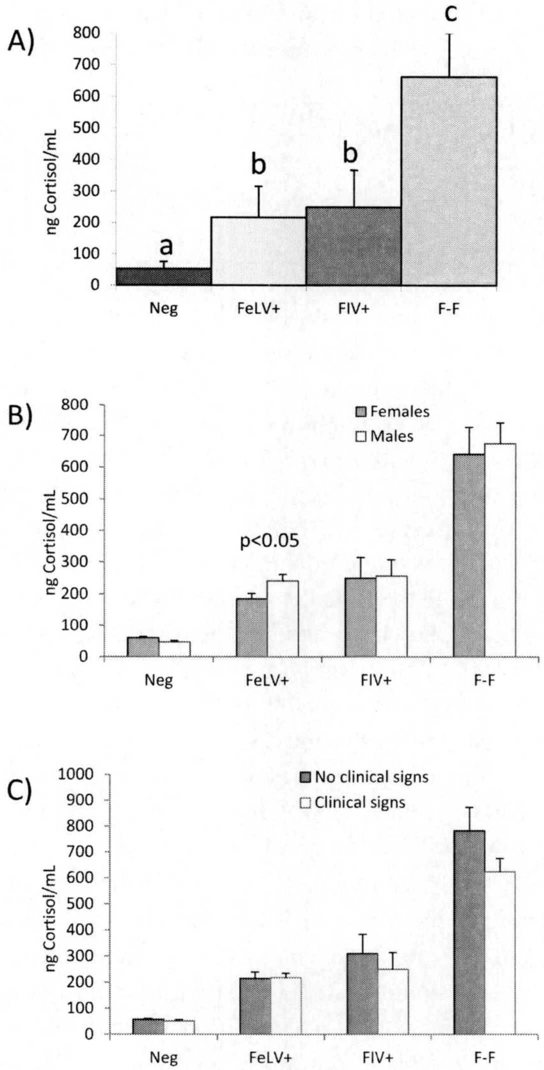

Figure 3. Concentration of plasma cortisol in retrovirus-infected and non-infected cats. A) Concentration of cortisol in each study group; groups identified with the same letter do not have statistically significant differences between them, while groups with different letters have statistically significant differences ($p<0.05$) between them. B) Concentration of cortisol in each study group in relation to the sex of the cats. C) Concentration of cortisol in each study group in relation to the presence or absence of clinical signs in cats. Neg, non-infected cats; FeLV+, cats infected by FeLV; FIV+, cats infected by FIV; F-F, double infected cats.

Table 1. Concentration of cortisol and DHEA expressed in ng/mL in the four groups of cats considered. SD, standard deviation

	Cortisol (SD)	DHEA (SD)	Cortisol/DHEA
Negative	53 (4.24)	10.4 (0.46)	5.1
FeLV-positive	213 (17.5)	5.9 (0.62)	36.3
FIV-positive	217 (58.4)	5.0 (0.34)	43.1
FeLV and FIV-positive	662 (76.7)	1.8 (0.62)	358.8

DHEA is the main and most abundant adrenal androgen. It has been associated with multiple beneficial effects for the body, though its mechanism of action and whether the hormone itself or its subproducts are responsible for these effects is still greatly unknown. Conceivably, the effects would be exerted through binding to an array of nuclear and cell surface receptors, and acting as a neurosteroid. DHEA is thought to interfere with the biosynthesis of cortisol through the enzyme 11β-HSD1, which has been suggested to be involved in the anti-glucocorticoid effects of DHEA (Muller et al., 2006), antagonizing by this route the immune suppressive effects of GCs.

DHEA has been shown to inhibit the replication of HIV-1 *in vitro* (Henderson et al., 1992) and to inhibit the reactivation of the latency of HIV-1 (Yang et al., 1993). Low levels of this hormone would be associated with a higher risk of progression to the most severe form of AIDS. The inhibitory effect of DHEA on FIV replication has also been shown (Bradley et al., 1995; Pedersen et al., 2003). In fact, DHEA has been administered to FIV-infected cats (Pedersen et al., 2003) and to patients with AIDS (Abrams et al., 2007; Rabkin et al., 2006) to boost their cell mediated immunity. In women, DHEA levels are higher than in men, and it could be a mechanism to explain the higher progression rate to AIDS in men than in women. In general, the reduction in $CD4^+$ cell counts is associated with the decrease in the levels of both DHEA and its derivate, DHEAS in both infected men and women (Chittiprol et al., 2009; Christeff et al., 2000; Laudat et al., 1995; Maingat et al., 2012; Schifitto et al., 2000; Zapanti et al., 2008). The increase in the cortisol/DHEA ratio could contribute, at least in part, to two fundamental facts in the pathogenesis of the HIV infection: the altered cytokine pattern and immune function, and the critical loss of lean body mass in patients with wasting syndrome. Lipodistrophy correlates with serum DHEA and increased cortisol/DHEA ratio, and with IFN-α levels in HIV-1-infected patients (Andersen et al., 2007; Christeff et al., 2000, 2002b; Norbiato et al., 2000; Zapanti et al., 2008).

The same cats as mentioned above were analyzed for the plasma or serum concentration of DHEA (Tejerizo et al., 2012). The values obtained are shown in Table 1. A similar trend to what is observed in HIV-1 infection could be seen in cats infected with FeLV or FIV. The concentration of plasma DHEA was significantly higher in the negative cats than in the infected cats, and in cats with monoinfection (either FIV or FeLV) than with dual infection. However, in our study the plasma concentration of DHEA in retrovirus-infected cats did not correlate with the presence or absence of clinical disease, unlike previously reported data on HIV infection (Christeff et al., 2000), but FIV-infected females had higher plasma levels of DHEA than males. This higher plasma levels of DHEA could be somehow involved in a greater survival of queens with respect to male cats that we detected earlier (Arjona et al., 2000). In general, it seems that the infection and disease stages are extremely important in the hormonal deregulation associated with retroviruses. Unfortunately, due to the highly dispersed origin of our samples, we could not do a follow-up of the animals, characterize in detail their clinical status, or analyze the stage of the infection at the time of blood collection. The wide range of possibilities associated with such non-specific clinical signs which characterize these infections, only allowed us to classify cats with and without clinical signs.

One of the most obvious consequences of the increase in plasma cortisol levels is the effect on the cytokine patterns. A shift from type-1 to type-2 cytokine production is detected in most HIV-1 patients during disease progression. This shift includes a defective production of IFN-γ, IL-2, and IL-12 along with the increased production of IL-4, IL-5, IL-6 and IL-10. GCs and IL-4 stimulate the differentiation of B lymphocytes into IgE-producing plasma cells, the concentration of which augments in HIV infection (Clerici et al., 2000).

MECHANISM OF CORTISOL DEREGULATION

The mechanisms by which viral infection causes this hormonal deregulation are still not clear and have been analyzed mostly in HIV infection. Although the mechanisms leading to adverse effects on HPA axis activity in HIV infection are not fully understood, several lines of evidence suggest that a number of mechanisms may be involved, including homologies in molecular structures of various mediators of neuroendocrine activity and

HIV-related structures, HIV as a chronic stress model, and virus-induced toxic factors (Kumar et al., 2002).

A possibility could be that the immune response, activated to fight the virus, triggers several signaling pathways, mainly mediated by cytokines, which could interfere with the regulatory mechanisms of the neuroendocrine system (*indirect regulation*). On the other hand, the infection could be interfering with the endocrine routes in a direct way, through the interaction of the virus or its products with elements of the neuroendocrine system (for example, infection in the hypothalamus) (*direct regulation*). In both cases, the virus could also interact with the end components of the HPA axis, the adrenal glands, without affecting the other elements of the endocrine control. Data supporting either route are discussed below.

In the case of *indirect regulation*, mediated by the activation of the immune response, it has been shown that both FeLV and FIV infections lead to an increase in the expression of proinflammatory cytokines such as IL-1, IL-6, TNFα (Gómez et al., 2011; Lawrence et al., 1995; Peterson and Chesebro, 2006; Robert-Tissot et al., 2011), and can activate the HPA axis (Besedovsky and del Rey, 1996). This activation would lead to an increase in levels of circulating GCs as has been shown for HIV-1 (Clerici et al., 2000; George and Bhangoo, 2013). Alterations in the production of adrenal steroids and a complex pattern of deregulation in cytokine profiles accompany the progression of HIV infection (Clerici et al., 2000). It has been observed that in some viral infections (*eg*.: produced by cytomegalovirus, or Newcastle disease paramyxovirus) the presence of certain cytokines, such as IL-1 or IL-6, can be decisive for the activation of this circuit (Dunn and Vickers, 1994; Ruzek et al., 1997). Although these interactions are known in acute phase responses, it has not been determined what happens really in cases of continuous stimulation or in conditions of chronic pathologies, as could be the case of retroviral infections. Numerous observations endorse also the hypothesis of a *direct regulation* of the HPA axis by the virus or its proteins. These viruses and other related viruses, such as HIV, are known to cross the brain-blood barrier and invade the central nervous system (CNS) and cause neurological damages in the host (Carmichael et al., 2002; Fletcher et al., 2008, 2009; Koirala et al., 2000; Podell et al., 2000; Ryan et al., 2005; Vahlenkamp et al., 1999). The presence of the virus within the control centers could alter the activation routes of the hypothalamus-pituitary axis and modify the endocrine regulation of the HPA axis, leading to the production of anomalous hormone levels. In this sense, the presence of FeLV or its proteins in the hypothalamus has been linked to an endocrine deregulation, affecting the concentrations of growth hormone (Tshikuka et al., 1992) or the HPA circuit in general (Wang and Teng, 1994). Cytoplasmic viral antigens have been detected by indirect immunofluorescence assays in the fibers of hypothalamic preoptic region of FeLV-infected cats (Wang and Teng, 1994). A similar dysfunction could be due to the presence of FIV in these regulating elements. The neurological damages associated to the lentiviral infection are partly mediated by the neurotoxicity of the envelope protein of the virus (Johnston et al., 2002; Power et al., 2004). Data supporting this are: a) It has been shown that the expression of HIV gp120 in the brain, frequently detected in AIDS patients, increases the concentrations of CRH, ACTH and cortisol (Costa et al., 2000; Raber et al., 1996); b) Treatment with GCs worsens the neurological damage produced by this viral protein (Brooke and Sapolsky, 2000, 2002); c) In connection with the indirect effects mentioned in the previous paragraph, encephalitis associated to the infection by HIV leads to an increase in the levels of proinflammatory cytokines, such as IL-1, IL-6, and TNFα (Persidsky et al., 1997). Altogether, these data could endorse the capacity of FeLV or FIV of interacting directly with neuroendocrine mechanisms of regulation.

Another possibility is the direct interaction between the *adrenal gland* and the retrovirus or cytokines secreted as a result of the infection, independently of initial elements of the regulating axis. This would induce a direct increase in the levels of GCs without the involvement of the hypothalamus or the pituitary gland. This has been demonstrated in other viral infections, such as infections by murine cytomegalovirus (Ruzek et al., 1997) or by Newcastle disease virus (Smith et al., 1982), and in certain cases of sepsis and chronic and autoimmune diseases. Mechanisms involving other elements are also possible. For example, in some HIV-positive patients who develop AIDS, the ability of cortisol to bind the cortisol binding globulin (CBG), responsible for the transportation of the hormone to its target tissues, is affected. This could limit even more the functional ability of the GCs (Martin et al., 1992).

The result of this inability of CBG is a continued activation of HPA axis and an increasing concentration of GCs unable to control their own production by feedback mechanisms.

CONSEQUENCES OF THE CORTISOL UNBALANCE

The neuroendocrine axis is indisputably essential to recover the basal homeostasis of the host after the infection (Ruzek et al., 1997; Silverman et al., 2005). Both FeLV and FIV could have acquired certain evolutionary advantage when interacting with this system, because they could benefit from the immunosuppression associated to its chronic activation. In addition, FIV and FeLV would also benefit from the shift of the Th1- to the Th2-type response mediated by cytokines in response to GCs. This shift involves an excess of antibodies and a weak cellular response. An effective defense against these intracellular pathogens needs to be mediated by a strong cellular immunity.

In our study, the cortisol levels were significantly higher and DHEA levels were significantly lower in double-infected cats than in cats with monoviral infection. Two hypotheses could explain this observation. If some infected animals were especially immune depressed, due to a greater alteration in the cortisol/DHEA ratio, they could be more susceptible to other pathogens, including the other retrovirus (FIV in the case of initial FeLV infection and vice versa). A second possibility could be that the infection by a second retrovirus would affect more markedly the concentration of both hormones. As we discussed previously, in the cortisol/DHEA balance it is difficult to differentiate the cause from the effect and to determine whether the unbalance is due to the retroviral infection or it derives from the physiological system of stress against infection. It has been proposed that GR could be a key protein exploited by HIV at multiple levels to ensure its pathogenic success (Hapgood and Tomasicchio, 2010). Besides the evident direct effect on the HPA axis of the viral infection and the immune system triggered by it, other conditions, concomitant to the infection, such as pain, weakening, or physiological stress may also participate actively in the activation of the HPA axis, increasing the GCs levels and making it even more difficult to establish the role of each component in the endocrinal regulation.

Treatment with Corticoids

The interaction between retrovirus and the HPA axis has serious *clinical implications*. GCs are routinely included in therapeutic protocols for retrovirosis as depressants of the immune response to revert the complications associated to the retroviral infection, such as neuropathies, renal disease, skin exanthema, gut inflammation, reactivation of a clinical toxoplasmosis (Lin et al., 1992), Burkitt lymphoma or pneumonia by *Pneumocystis carinii* (Barr et al., 2000). Treatment with GCs, such as dexamethasone or prednisolone, could be detrimental for an already immune suppressed host, in spite of their powerful anti-inflammatory effect. In these cases a therapeutic intervention aimed to diminish the endogenous levels of GCs would be more effective. The detrimental effect of steroid therapy has been shown in FeLV- or FIV-infected cats. Cats treated with GCs before being infected experimentally with FeLV lost their natural resistance to persistent viremia (Rojko et al., 1988). In the case of FIV, it has been shown that the administration of GCs increases the levels of viral ARN in plasma (Barr et al., 2000). Therefore, the effects of GC administration should be a factor to consider when choosing the most suitable therapy for retroviral infection. In addition, it has been reported that antiretroviral therapy may increase cortisol levels in HIV-1 infected patients (Collazos et al., 2004). However, this does not seem to be the case in FIV-infected treated cats (at least with zidovudine) (Gómez et al., 2011).

In conclusion, the possible alterations of the levels of cortisol during the infection by feline retroviruses have not received so far the attention they deserve. According to our data, concentration of cortisol is greatly increased in FIV, FeLV or FIV and FeLV-infected animals. The fact that in double-infected animals levels are three times higher than in the single infection suggests a different mechanism of action of cortisol for both viruses. It is difficult to know whether the host activates mechanisms to increase the levels of cortisol to fight the retroviral infection, or FIV and FeLV induce this increase. Undoubtedly, elevated cortisol levels have an impact on the feline homeostasis, as it is an immunosuppressor, acts on innate immunity, lymphocyte proliferation and cytotoxicity and antigen presentation. Most importantly, it alters the cytokine expression promoting the shift of Th1 to Th2 immune responses. All these are effects of cortisol at the organic level; the next question to address is what the implications at the cellular level are.

EFFECT OF CORTISOL AT THE CELLULAR LEVEL

One of the parameters in which cortisol could be affecting at the cellular level would be apoptosis. Steroid hormones have been reported previously to induce apoptosis of lymphocytes of FeLV-infected cats (Rojko et al., 1979), FIV-infected cats (Hofmann-Lehmann et al., 1998), or FeLV-infected cells in culture (Tejerizo et al., 2005). To determine whether cortisol would also produce a similar effect, FeLV- or FIV-infected cells were exposed to serial dilutions of cortisol or dexamethasone (a potent synthetic glucocorticoid) (10^{-3}M to 10^{-12}M). After 24 h or 48 h, cells were stained with Annexin V-Fluos (Annex) and propidium iodide (PI) to differentiate apoptotic cells (Annex +, PI-) from dead cells (Annex+ or -, PI+) and evaluated by flow cytometry. Cell-free supernatants were used to determine RT Activity and FeLV-p27 or FIV-p24 as described by Tejerizo et al. (2005).

In general, both cortisol and dexamethasone induced apoptosis of FeLV-infected cells at high concentrations (mostly 10^{-3}M) after 24 h and 48 h exposure, but the effect was noticeable in a wide range of concentrations, up till at least 10^{-7}M (Figure 5A, 5C, 5E, 5G). The effect of these GCs on FIV-infected cells was less marked. After 48 h exposure to cortisol and dexamethasone, increased apoptosis was observed in the range between 10^{-5}M to 10^{-8}M (Figure 6A, 6C, 6E, 6G). The ability of the GCs to induce apoptosis and regulate proliferation has been described previously in a multitude of cell types, including cells of the immune system (Amsterdam and Sasson, 2002; Webb et al., 2003) and in relation to tumor progression involving c-Myb (Sarvaiya et al., 2012).

In regards to feline retroviruses, although FeLV and FIV have been shown to induce apoptosis in lymphoid cells (Bull et al., 2004; Rojko and Kociba, 1991; Rojko et al., 1988, 1979, 1992; Sprague et al., 2010; Tompkins et al., 2002), the phenomenon has not been analyzed extensively in the presence of GCs. Barr et al. (2000) detected in *in vivo* studies a decline in lymphocyte subpopulations in FIV-infected cats treated with prednisolone, without significant alterations in the CD4/CD8 ratio.

The mechanisms involved in this decline were not examined and other processes related to hormone action may be involved. Other steroid hormones induce apoptosis. For example, the group of Hoffmann-Lehmann found differences in the apoptosis rate in males and females infected by FIV, and these correlated to the blood levels of 17β-estradiol and progesterone (Hoffmann-Lehmann et al., 1998). The apoptotic activity of both 17β-estradiol and progesterone has also been shown on FeLV-infected cells (Tejerizo et al., 2005). In other viruses, GCs may protect from apoptosis. Thus, it has been shown that GCs improve the survival of HIV-infected T cells by repressing apoptosis (Lu et al., 1995). However, other studies have shown that cortisol and HIV-1 gp120 act synergistically to induce apoptosis of lymphocytes from normal donors as demonstrated by DNA ladder formation and other techniques, and this was more significant in the $CD4^+$ population than in the CD47 population (Clerici et al., 2000; Nair et al., 2000). This GC-induced apoptosis of mature T lymphocytes may be responsible, at least in part, of the pathogenesis of HIV-1. Because (1) Th1 but not Th2 undergo rapid apoptosis upon antigen-stimulation, and (2) Th2 clones preferentially survive in *in vitro* cell cultures, the progressive shift from type-1 to type-2 cytokine production observed in HIV infection could be at least partially provoked by the increase in the production of cortisol and the reduction of DHEA (Clerici et al., 2000).

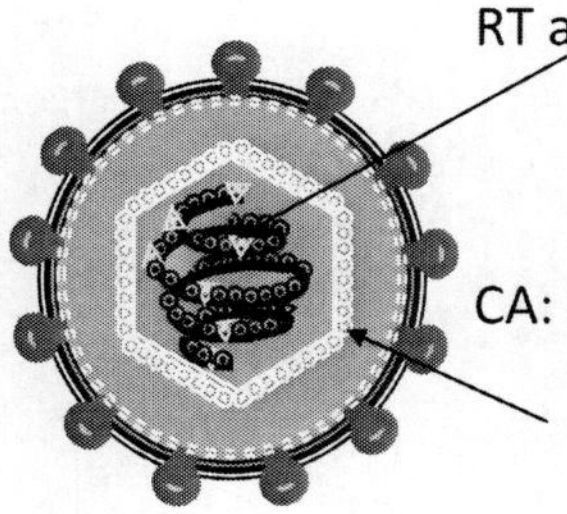

Figure 4. Different approaches for determining the effect of cortisol on the expression of viral particles.

In conclusion, it seems that GCs play a role in apoptosis. What consequences does this have for the retroviral cycle? Apoptosis (also called programmed cell death or PCD) is a type of cell death in which enzymes break down the cytoskeleton of the cell, upon which the cytoplasm becomes dense, with the organelles tightly packed. Characteristically, chromatin condenses and the nuclear envelope breaks, as well as the DNA (when run in a gel, a typical ladder of DNA fragments of different size may be seen). All this happens while the cell plasma membrane remains apparently intact, though its chemical composition is modified, and usually "blebs" are seen protruding from the cell. Lastly, the cell breaks down into vesicles, the apoptotic bodies. The modifications of the plasma membrane may have important consequences on the viral cycle of retroviruses, including FIV and FeLV.

Two parameters are especially useful to study the effect of cortisol on the viral cycle and whether apoptosis plays a role in this effect: RT activity and the amount of capsid protein in the extracellular environment. RT activity measures the presence of infective viral particles in the supernatant (Marozsan et al., 2004; Niermann and Buehring, 1997), under the assumption that only infective viral particles will have active RT. Unlike RT activity, the amount of capsid protein p27 of FeLV (FeLV-p27), and less markedly of p24 of FIV (FIV-p24), in the supernatant is not considered representative of the presence of viable particles (Figure 4). For unknown reasons, an undetermined percentage of the viral capsid proteins synthesized by some retrovirus is not incorporated into viable viral particles, and is released as free antigen or defective particles (Rojko et al., 1996, 1992; Jarrett, 2001; Marozsan et al., 2004).

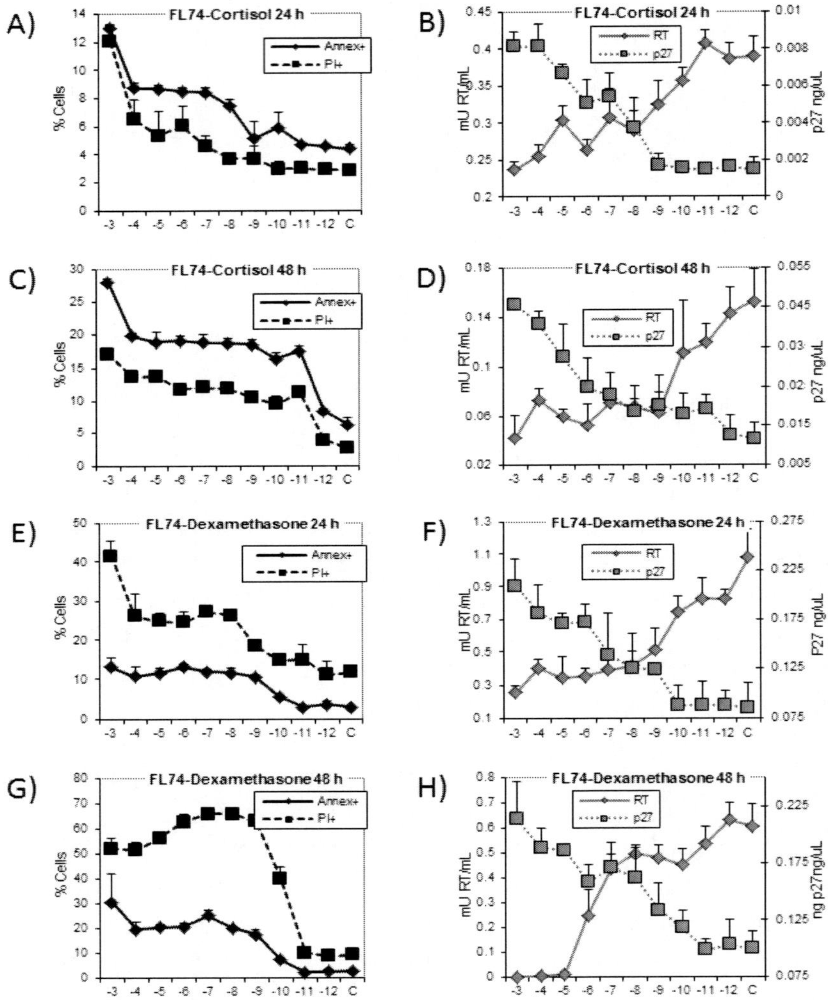

Figure 5. Effect of cortisol (A-D) and dexamethasone (E-H) on cellular viability and RT activity (mU/mL) and FeLV-p27 presence in the supernatant of treated chronically FeLV-infected cells (FL74) after 24 (A, B, E, F) or 48 (C, D, G, H) hours of exposure. Apoptotic cells are identified by the positive reaction to Annexin V (Annex+, PI-) while dead cells are identified by the positive reaction to PI (PI+). RT, RT activity.

EFFECT OF GLUCOCORTICOIDS ON FELV-INFECTED CELLS

Interestingly, GCs had an opposite effect on FeLV-infected cells and on FIV-infected cells (Figures 5 and 6). In FeLV-infected cells, at high concentrations of both cortisol and dexamethasone, there was a high concentration of FeLV-p27 detected in the supernatant, which decreased as the hormone concentration decreased (Figure 5B, 5D, 5F, 5H). These high concentrations of FeLV-p27 could not be due only to cellular lysis (which would indeed promote the release of p27), as the results obtained when adding a lysis buffer were similar to controls with just culture medium. Thus, it could be assumed that cortisol and dexamethasone enhance the synthesis and release of FeLV-p27, independent from cellular viability, increasing its secretion. Contrariwise, the lowest RT activity values were invariably detected at the highest GCs concentrations (10^{-3}M) and at around 10^{-11}M they were comparable (in general) to that in the controls without hormone (Figure 5B, 5D, 5F, 5H). When cells were completely lysed using lysis buffer, high RT activity values were found in the supernatant, similar to controls, suggesting that simple lysis would free viable viral particles from cells. However, at 10^{-3}M of either cortisol or dexamethasone, even when cell counts and viability were very low (indicating high cell death), RT activity was considerably less than when using lysis buffer. This observation seems to suggest that in the presence of cortisol or dexamethasone cells might have died through a process of apoptosis, which might suppress the release of viable viral particles to the extracellular environment, possibly by alterations in the plasma membrane, thus presenting an inverse relationship between both variables (apoptosis and viral shedding). Taken together, these data may mean that high concentrations of GCs, such as cortisol or dexamethasone, enhance apoptosis of FeLV-infected cells. This would hamper the budding of infective particles (a parameter quantified by RT activity) and the increased protein synthesis would not culminate to form infective viral particles; thus, high concentrations of GCs would be protective for the cat. The effect of GCs on FeLV-infected cells agrees with results with 17β-estradiol and progesterone (Tejerizo et al., 2005).

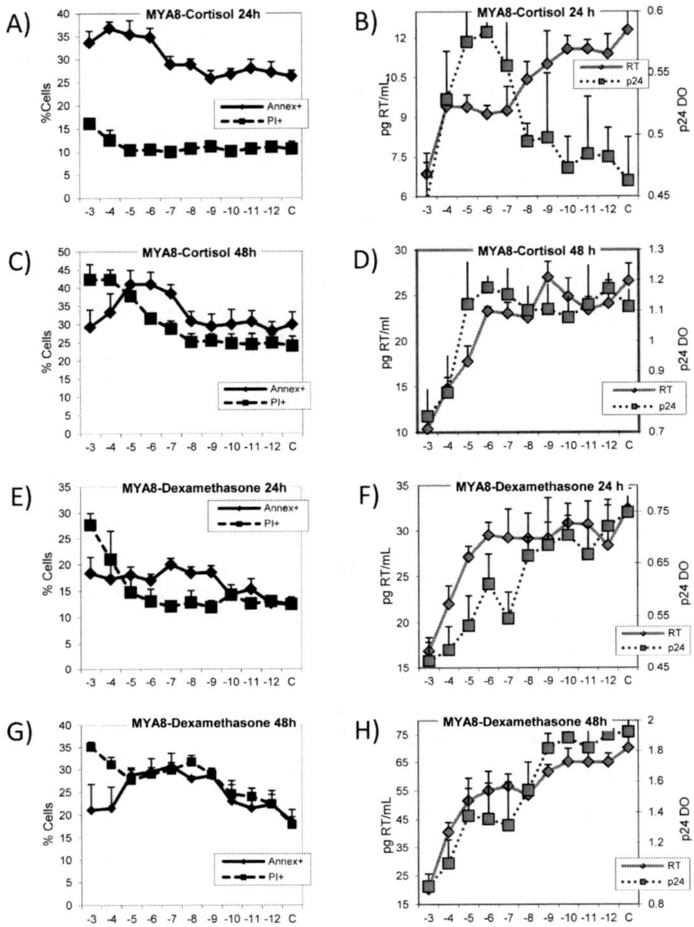

Figure 6. Effect of cortisol (A-D) and dexamethasone (E-H) on cellular viability and RT activity and FIV-p24 presence in the supernatant of treated FIV-infected cells (MYA-8) after 24 (A, B, E, F) or 48 (C, D, G, H) hours of exposure. Apoptotic cells are identified by the positive reaction to Annexin V (Annex+, PI-) while dead cells are identified by the positive reaction to PI (PI+). RT, RT activity.

Effect of Glucocorticoids on FIV-Infected Cells

Contrarily to what was observed in FeLV-infected cells, the expression of viral proteins in FIV-infected cells (as quantified by the presence of FIV-p24 in the supernatant) was repressed when these cells were exposed to high concentrations of either cortisol or dexamethasone, though RT activity levels were similar in FeLV- and in FIV-infected cells (Figure 6). In the case of FIV, other additional mechanisms must exist that also influence RT activity, because the relationship between both parameters was not as homogeneous in FIV- as in FeLV-infected cultures and in some cases there was a decrease of RT activity without marked alterations in the rate of apoptosis. The greater biological complexity of FIV, mainly associated to the presence of regulatory proteins (encoded by *vif*, *rev* and *orf2*), could be responsible for the decrease of RT activity, somewhat independently from apoptosis.

Our findings do not agree with those reported in other studies. Barr et al. (2000) detected both an increase of the RT activity in PBMCs of prednisolone-treated FIV-infected cats, and an increase of plasma viremia in these same cats when compared to non-treated FIV-infected cats. An increase in the HIV RT activity was also found in cultures of lymphoid and monocytic cell lines incubated in the presence of cortisol and dexamethasone (Soudeyns et al., 1993). Niermann and Buehring (1997) also found an increase in RT activity of BLV (not a lentivirus, but also encoding a regulatory protein) in cultures of epithelial lung cells exposed to dexamethasone. According to these observations, it seems that GCs would favor viral replication and, therefore, the development of the infection, contrasting with our results, in which it appears that GCs inhibit the formation of infective viral particles. However, differences may be explained when analyzing assay conditions. For example, in the case of BLV, RT activity was studied in cultures selected for their resistance to GCs (Niermann and Buehring, 1997).

In previous studies with feline retroviruses (Barr et al., 2000), studies were done on cell populations isolated from infected animals treated with GCs, without the *in vitro* addition of GCs. In this case, other secondary factors derived from the immunosuppression induced by this hormone may play a relevant role.

It could be argued that the physiological concentration of cortisol in healthy cats is in the range of 10^{-8}M, and even in infected cats it is not higher than 10^{-7}M, concentrations far lower than those in which the most evident effects of hormones were observed. However, in the course of the experiments described here, it was also observed that the "freshness" of the cells affected the results, and cells which had been passaged 7-10 days before the beginning of the experiment at extreme conditions (1:40) were affected by the hormones at concentrations far lower (10^{-8}M) than cells passed 1:5 two or three days before the beginning of the experiment. It may be assumed that circulating lymphocytes can correspond to this "aged" population rather than to the "fresh" population, as renovation from the bone marrow does not happen as fast as in culture media *in vitro*. Thus, circulating lymphocytes would be more affected by lower concentrations of hormones.

From the results presented above it became evident that GCs affected the presence of feline retroviruses in the extracellular environment. The effect was both through indirect and direct mechanisms. Indirectly, by activating cellular apoptosis, GCs may suppress budding of virions to the extracellular environment. This would benefit the cat, and is more obvious in the case of FeLV.

Glucocorticoids also had an effect on viral protein expression, which was the opposite in FeLV and in FIV. The increased expression of FeLV-p27 and decreased of FIV-p24 at high doses of cortisol or dexamethasone suggest that these GCs had a direct effect on viral expression, stimulating or repressing the transcriptional ability of these feline retroviruses. Together with the sharp increase in the serum levels of cortisol detected in infected cats, these data suggest an important role for GCs in the pathogenesis of FeLV and FIV.

Effect of Cortisol at the Molecular Level

Few studies have been undertaken to determine the effect of steroid hormones directly on the expression of feline retroviruses. The molecular mechanism of action of cortisol, as in the case of other steroids, involves binding to intracellular molecules. Cortisol is able to diffuse through the cell membrane into the cytoplasm, where it binds to the glucocorticoid receptor (GR). Homodimer GR-cortisol complexes are translocated to the nucleus, where they bind specific DNA sequences called glucocorticoid responsive elements (GRE) (or more broadly, hormone responsive elements or HRE) and activate gene transcription (Figure 7). A second mechanism involves the binding of GR-cortisol to NF-κB or AP-1 factors or to the DNA binding sites (called transcription binding sites or TBS) for them, to repress them from transactivating target genes. These two mechanisms are called transactivation and transrepression, respectively.

HRE are responsible for the biological effects of cortisol, which depend also on the type of cell exposed to the steroid. For example, when GR-cortisol complexes cross the nuclear membrane of Th cells, they bind GRE which transactivate the IL-4, IL-10 or IL-13 genes and differentiate the lymphocyte into a Th2 cell. The GRE sequence has been identified to be TGTTCT, and is common for glucocorticoids, progesterone, androgens and mineralcorticoids.

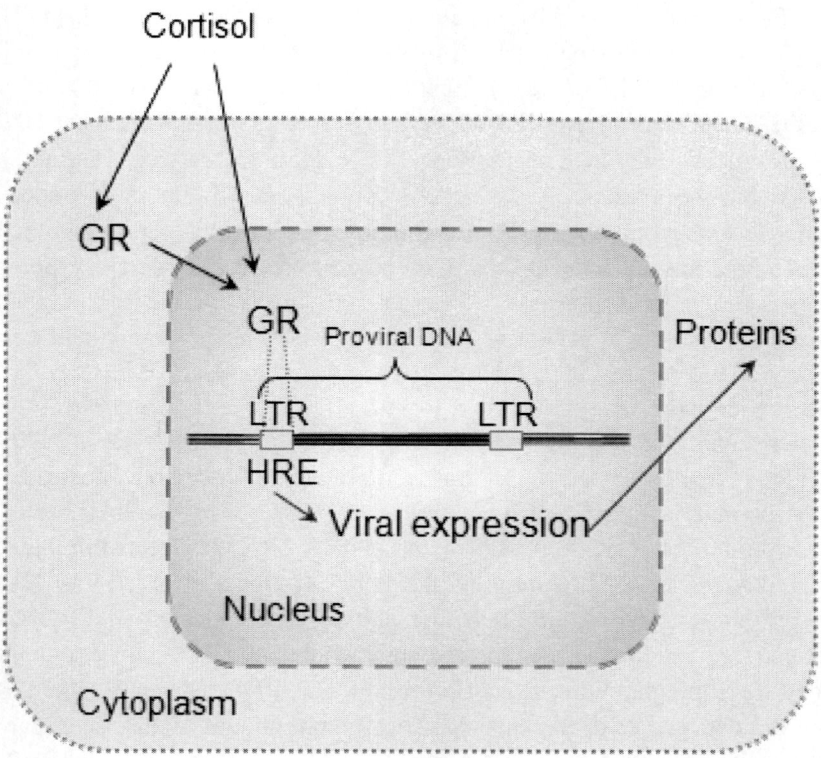

Figure 7. Direct mechanism of protein expression transactivation by cortisol. Due to its lipophilic nature, cortisol may freely cross cellular membranes to bind its receptors (GR), which are in the cytoplasm or in the nucleus. The complex cortisol-GR crosses the nuclear membrane and is recognized by specific DNA sequences called glucocorticoid responsive elements (GRE). GREs have been found in the LTR of several retroviruses. The recognition of the cortisol-GR complex by these GRE in the LTR triggers transcription which culminates in the expression of viral proteins.

The first indication that steroids could affect the expression of retroviruses stems from the 60s when Smoller et al. (1961) observed inclusion bodies in the cytoplasm of cortisol-treated mammary tumors produced by the mouse mammary tumor virus (MMTV).

It was found that when dexamethasone (a potent synthetic glucocorticoid), progesterone, testosterone or mineralcorticoids were added to the culture medium of cells infected by MMTV, there was an increase in the viral RNA (Ringold et al., 1975; Smoller et al., 1961), suggesting that GCs could stimulate replication and expression of the virus. Later, the presence of a GRE was identified in the genome of MMTV (Majors and Varmus, 1983; McGrath,

1971; Payvar et al., 1983; Slater et al., 1989; Stewart et al., 1988). This GRE is a sequence 75 to 195 base pair (bp) long mapped to the 5' long terminal repeats region (LTR, Figure 7). LTRs are sequences which flank the viral genome in the state of provirus (*i.e.* when it is integrated in the host DNA), playing crucial roles in transcription. The relationship between steroids and MMTV has been intensely studied, becoming one of the most important models for understanding genome regulation. The effect of steroids directing transcription has also been shown in other retroviruses such as Moloney murine sarcoma virus, murine endogenous retroviruses, bovine leukemia virus, porcine endogenous retroviruses, and simian and human immunodeficiency viruses (Diallo et al., 2000; Ghosh, 1992; Lan et al., 1984; Miksicek et al., 1986; Niermann and Buehring, 1997; Quinn and Langford, 2001; Ramakrishnan and Robins, 1997; Rousseau, 1984; Russo et al., 1999). Mutations in this site in several retroviruses induce the decrease of transcriptional activity when exposed to GCs, proving their role in transcription (Nishigaki et al., 1997). In FeLV, a GRE was located in the LTR (GRE: nt. -184 to -179) (Fulton et al., 1990; Nishigaki et al., 1997). To the best of our knowledge, no such element has been located in FIV. GCs-mediated regulation has also been demonstrated in DNA viruses, such as herpesvirus and papillomavirus (Poreba et al., 1998; Slater et al., 1989). However, data and studies related specifically to feline retroviruses are scarce.

In order to determine whether cortisol or dexamethasone would have an effect on FIV and FeLV transcriptional activity, their LTR was cloned into pEGFP-1 vector (Clontech) which does not contain any promoter of itself. Plasmids were transfected into CrFK cells and cells were treated with 10^{-3}M to 10^{-11}M of either cortisol or dexamethasone. Controls included cells transfected but not treated with glucocorticoid (C), and cells transfected with the empty plasmid (pEGFP). The expression of EGFP was quantified by flow cytometry 24 h after treating transfected cells with cortisol or dexamethasone.

In addition, EGFP allowed following the efficiency of transfection and the state of the cell population by fluorescence microscopy, locating and characterizing specifically cells based on their expression levels.

In the case of the plasmid containing the LTR of FeLV, higher expression of EGFP was observed at the higher concentrations of both cortisol and dexamethasone (Figure 8A and 8B), while in the case of the plasmid containing the LTR of FIV, the opposite was observed (Figure 8C and 8D). This parallels the findings of the quantification of the capsid protein in the supernatant upon the exposure to the glucocorticoids.

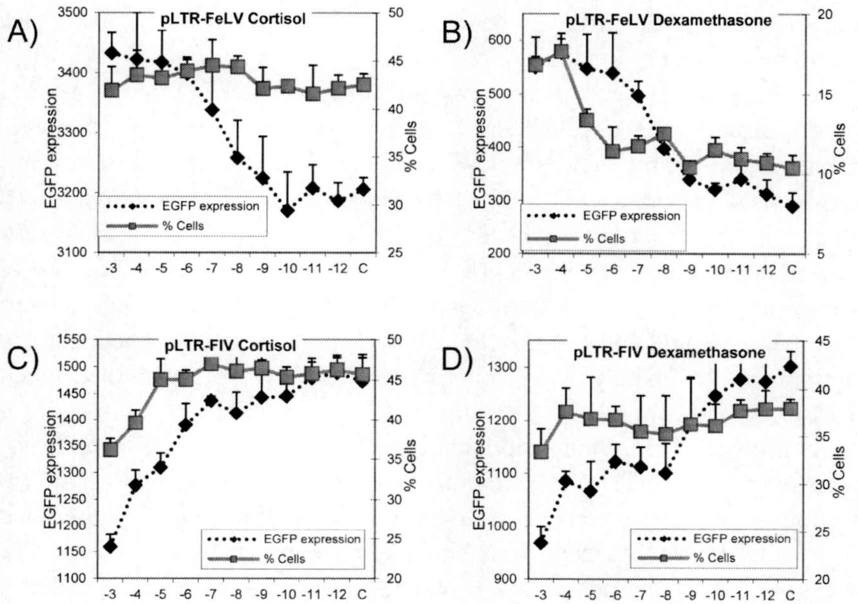

Figure 8. Effect of cortisol (A, C) and dexamethasone (B, D) on the expression and on the percentage of cells expression EGFP in CrFK cultures transfected with a plasmid containing the LTR of FeLV (Rickard A strain) (A, B) or the LTR of FIV (Glasgow 8 strain) (C, D) after 24 hours of incubation.

We may conclude that both FIV and FeLV seem to have a functional GRE, as the expression of EGFP varies with the different concentration of cortisol or dexamethasone.

Our data on FeLV increased expression of EGFP and FeLV-p27 at high concentrations of GCs associated to the GRE sequence present in the LTR coincide with those obtained by Nishigaki et al. (1997). These researchers showed that mutations in the LTR-FeLV GRE region led to a decline in the transcriptional activity in both feline and human lymphoid cell lines and in CrFK fibroblasts. In addition, this region is highly conserved in different clones of FeLV (Fulton et al., 1990), which suggests its probable involvement in viral regulation.

As the expression of FeLV viral proteins could increase in the presence of GCs, and cortisol concentration is significantly increased in FeLV-infected cats, viral genomes which take advantage of this could have been selected along the evolution to maximize their transmission and to escape the immune response. The observations of Rojko et al. (1979) would support this hypothesis. They showed that FeLV-infected cats treated with prednisolone lost their natural resistance to persistent viremia, *i.e.* treatment with GCs favored the survival of the virus.

On the other hand, the response to cortisol via LTR could play an additional role in the development of tumor processes, strongly associated with oncogenic viruses such as FeLV, by the insertional activation of different protooncogenes (Dudley et al., 2002; Morrison et al., 1995). The proviral LTR sequence carrying a functional GRE could be inserted close to oncogenes, providing them with certain degree of sensitivity to hormonal activation (Beato et al., 1989). An increase of GCs, associated with factors such as stress or pregnancy, could thus trigger an adjacent protooncogene, leading to its expression and ultimately to the abnormal growth of the cell and tumorigenic processes.

Contrarily to FeLV, transcriptional activity directed by the FIV-LTR was suppressed at high GC concentrations, coinciding with the results of the detection of FIV capsid protein (FIV-p24) in the supernatant. In the case of HIV-1, a GRE site has been found in its *vif* sequence, which favors viral replication when exposed to GCs (Soudeyns et al., 1993). In FIV, which is also a lentivirus, the existence of this GRE site or any other GC binding consensus sequence in the viral LTR has not been described. Data shown above suggest that the effect of cortisol would be transrepression as explained at the beginning of this section, instead of transactivation, not involving a GRE but rather other cellular pathways such as NF-κB or AP-1 as described below.

Despite a growing body of evidence on the relationships between pathogens and GCs, little is known yet on the effect of these steroids on viruses associated with immunodeficiency syndromes. A regulatory effect of the GCs on different retroviruses has been reported. The results obtained for lentiviruses, mainly HIV, are heterogeneous. However, they all agree in accepting the involvement of GCs in its pathogenesis. GCs have been described to both activate and repress the expression of HIV, and some researchers have shown the presence of several GREs in its sequence, both in the LTR and in intragenic regions (Ghosh, 1992; Kino et al., 2000; Mitra et al., 1995; Russo et al., 1999; Soudeyns et al., 1993; Vanitharani et al., 2001). In general, it seems clear the possibility of a differential regulation depending on the cell type and the intracellular factors specific for each cellular lineage (Kino et al., 2000; Mitra et al., 1995).

It is becoming increasingly apparent that the mechanisms of action of the GCs are more varied from what until recently has been believed. Currently, intracellular processes based on the direct regulation of transcription (specific binding of the GC-GR or GR, to TBS), in addition to the classic mechanism, are recognized. These processes do not involve the complex GC-GR, although it is believed that they do require the glucocorticoid receptor (GR), and involve a number of interactions with different biochemical routes.

Our results show that GCs inhibit transcription directed by the FIV-LTR in lymphoid lines and fibroblasts. These data coincide with those published for HIV by other researchers (Kino et al., 2000; Mitra et al., 1995). In these cases, the GCs effect appears to be mediated by GREs located in different positions within the LTR, mainly at the site +15 to +20 (Mitra et al., 1995), but there is no agreement about the functionality of the remaining sites. The LTR region of FIV does not present the GRE consensus sequence, which challenges an explanation based on this interaction between the hormone and DNA. GCs could interact, either with yet unidentified similar viral sequences, and regulate replication by a direct mechanism, or with other cellular factors involved in the regulation of viral replication by an indirect mechanism.

The *direct mechanism* to explain the decreased transcriptional activity of the FIV-LTR in the presence of high GCs concentrations would involve the existence of sequences similar to a GRE overlapping a positive regulatory factor. The union of GR to this site would displace the binding of this second factor, thus interfering with its activating effect. Different DNA sequences could support this hypothesis (Figure 10B), such as the TTGACT sequence (nt -125 /-120), which overlaps with the AP-1 transcription factor binding site (nt -124/-118). Something similar could happen in the sequences TGTTTT (nt -51/-46) and TGTTCC (nt -46/-41), due to their proximity to the ATF transcription factors binding sites (nt -58/-53).

Mechanisms involving other cellular signaling molecules (*indirect regulation*) are currently considered to explain the transrepression observed when protein expression was decreased when FIV-infected cells (cellular experiments) or FIV LTR (molecular experiments) were exposed to increased concentrations of GCs.

AP-1 and ATF are important regions in the regulation of FIV and are involved in the basal promoter activity of the LTR (Chatterji et al., 2002; Ikeda et al., 1998; Inoshima et al., 1996; Murphy et al., 2014; de Parseval and Elder, 1999; Thompson et al., 1994). Ikeda et al. (1998) showed that the nuclear factors that bind specifically to AP-1 and ATF sites of the FIV-LTR are present in several cell lines, including the two used in our experiments (CrFK and MYA-1). However, while these factors have similar properties, they are not exactly the same in both lines. Deletion experiments showed that the promoter activity was reduced in the absence of any of these fragments (AP-1 or ATF); this decrease was even more evident in the case of a double deletion, suggesting cooperation in the mechanism of transcriptional regulation. Similar results were obtained with deletion mutants in sites AP-1, C/EBP and ATF in the FIV-LTR in the CrFK cell line (de Parseval and Elder, 1999). On the other hand, in the case of AP-1, this assumed competition with the hormone-receptor complex would not be decisive for the replication of the virus, as other studies have proven that its deletion does not completely inactivate the process (Miyazawa et al., 1993), although it could be slower (Inoshima et al., 1996). In the case of FeLV, AP-1 (which has four sites not represented in the FeLV-LTR, Figure 9A) has been involved in the opposite phenomenon as in FIV: transactivation. Activation of mitogen-activated protein kinases 1 and 2 (MEK1 and -2) by the LTR is an intermediate step in the FeLV LTR-mediated induction of AP-1 activity (Ghosh and Faller, 1999). This would agree with our results.

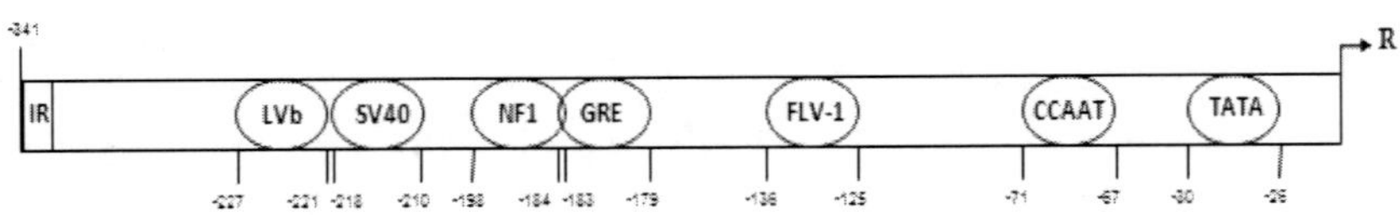

Figure 9. Schematic representation of the FeLV genome showing the most relevant transcription binding sites and their relative location.

It has also been shown that the AP-4 and AP-1 sites, which are quite close together (Figure 10A), can activate regulatory regions in a coordinated way (Mermod et al., 1988). This could be the case for the AP-4 (nt -134/-129) and AP-1 sites (nt -124/-118) of the FIV-LTR (de Parseval and Elder, 1999), where the efficient binding with their transcription factors could be affected by the presence of the GC-GR complex in a hypothetic adjacent GRE sequence. Lastly, and further supporting the importance of AP-1 and ATF sites, it is believed that the assumed transactivating Tat protein of FIV (ORF2) interacts with these sites of the LTR (de Parseval and Elder, 1999). The GC-GR complex could interfere with this interaction also by this mechanism.

Other proteins which have been thought to play a role in the repression of protein expression by GCs in retrovirus-infected cells are STAT (signal transducer and activator of transcription) 5, IκBα, nuclear factor I (NFI), and CCAAT displacement protein (CDP). STAT5 is activated when cells are exposed to IL-2 and GCs, inhibiting the GR transcriptional activity (Biola et al., 2001). In the case of IκBα, GC treatment increases the levels of this protein and reduces the amount of NF-κB, a strong activator of HIV-1 promoter, decreasing by this mechanism the transcription of HIV-1 (Kurata and Yamamoto, 1999). NFI sites have been shown to compete with the GC receptors for DNA binding, decreasing by this mechanism the effect of GCs in the MMTV model (Brüggemeier et al., 1990). This mechanism would be similar to that proposed by Zhu and Dudley (2002), in which CDP, expressed in high amounts in the naive mammary gland, would repress MMTV expression, playing a role in tumorigenesis.

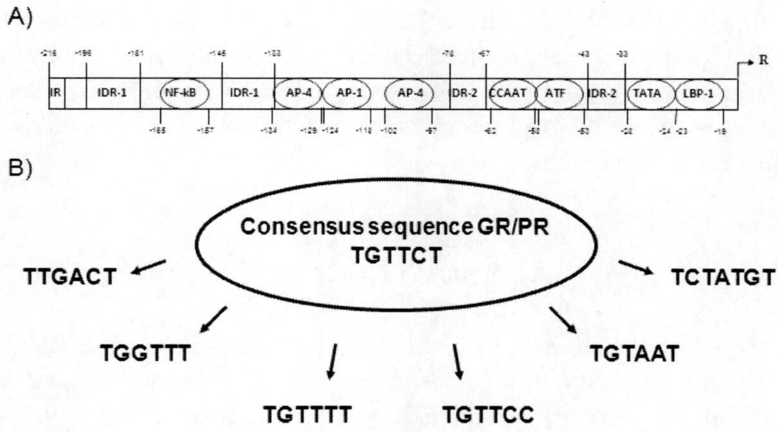

Figure 10. Transcription binding sites (TBS) in the LTR of FIV which could explain the transrepression observed when FIV-infected cells or FIV-LTR are exposed to high concentrations of GCs. A) Schematic representation of the FIV genome showing the most relevant TBS and their relative location. B) Alternative GRE sites in the FIV LTR. The consensus sequence for the glucocorticoids and progesterone (GR/PR) is shown in the oval.

Besides the effect through signaling molecules, other mechanisms of repression may be possible. For example, in HIV-1 LTR-independent pathways influenced by cytokine and GC through which HIV can maintain substantial levels of protein expression and virion production have been proposed (Kinter et al., 2001). These may involve Vpr (Mirani et al., 2002), which modulates host GR function to affect transcription of host genes, probably acting as a co-activator for the GR (Hapgood and Tomasicchio, 2010). Different isoforms of the glucocorticoid receptor have been recently described. Differential post-transcriptional processing and modification may give rise to different variants of this GR. It has been suggested that this variety of isoforms could lead to unique biological responses (Zhou and Cidlowski, 2005).

Although the differences between these isoforms are still greatly unknown, the presence of isoforms of GR in certain cell types may be involved in negative responses.

In summary, the results obtained and data reviewed support that glucocorticoids are important factors in the regulation of FeLV and FIV, through direct mechanisms, indirect mechanisms or, possibly, by the coordinated action of both. The increased plasma concentration of cortisol in FeLV-infected cats and the effect that high concentrations of cortisol have, increasing viral protein expression, should be taken into consideration when considering treating cats with immunosuppresants to treat FeLV-associated clinical signs. The role of glucocorticoids in feline retroviral infections is an exciting field which requires more studies.

ACKNOWLEDGMENT

The editorial assistance of David A. Bruhn is much appreciated. The authors thank Alejandro Esteller for his technical assistance in quantifying steroids and the veterinary practitioners who participated in this study. We are especially grateful to Gustavo Sanchez Visconti and the personnel of the Laboratorio de Analisis Veterinarios, as well as the staff of the Veterinary Clinic Hospital, for their kind collaboration. This study was supported by the Spanish Ministry of Science (AGL2002-02616) and UCM-920620. At the time, G.T. was a grantee of the Community of Madrid.

REFERENCES

Abrams, D. I., Shade, S. B., Couey, P., McCune, J. M., Lo, J., Bacchetti, P., Chang, B., Epling, L., Liegler, T., and Grant, R. M. (2007). Dehydroepiandrosterone (DHEA) effects on HIV replication and host immunity: a randomized placebo-controlled study. *AIDS Res. Hum. Retroviruses,* 23, 77–85.

Amsterdam, A., and Sasson, R. (2002). The anti-inflammatory action of glucocorticoids is mediated by cell type specific regulation of apoptosis. *Mol. Cell. Endocrinol.,* 189, 1–9.

Andersen, O., Pedersen, S. B., Svenstrup, B., Hansen, B. R., Paulsen, S. K., Rathje, G. S., Richelsen, B., Nielsen, J. O., Madsbad, S., Iversen, J., et al.

(2007). Circulating sex hormones and gene expression of subcutaneous adipose tissue oestrogen and alpha-adrenergic receptors in HIV-lipodystrophy: implications for fat distribution. *Clin. Endocrinol.,* (Oxf.) 67, 250–258.

Arjona, A., Escolar, E., Soto, I., Barquero, N., Martin, D., and Gomez-Lucia, E. (2000). Seroepidemiological survey of infection by feline leukemia virus and immunodeficiency virus in Madrid and correlation with some clinical aspects. *J. Clin. Microbiol., 38*, 3448–3449.

Arjona, A., Barquero, N., Doménech, A., Tejerizo, G., Collado, V. M., Toural, C., Martín, D., and Gomez-Lucia, E. (2007). Evaluation of a novel nested PCR for the routine diagnosis of feline leukemia virus (FeLV) and feline immunodeficiency virus (FIV). *J. Feline Med. Surg.*, 9, 14–22.

Barr, M. C., Huitron-Resendiz, S., Selway, D. R., Henriksen, S. J., and Phillips, T. R. (2000). Exogenous glucocorticoids alter parameters of early feline immunodeficiency virus infection. *J. Infect. Dis.,* 181, 576–586.

Beato, M., Chalepakis, G., Schauer, M., and Slater, E. P. (1989). DNA regulatory elements for steroid hormones. *J. Steroid Biochem.*, 32, 737–747.

Besedovsky, H. O., and del Rey, A. (1996). Immune-neuro-endocrine interactions: facts and hypotheses. *Endocr. Rev.*, 17, 64–102.

Bhathena, S. J. (2006). Relationship between fatty acids and the endocrine and neuroendocrine system. *Nutr. Neurosci.,* 9, 1–10.

Biola, A., Lefebvre, P., Perrin-Wolff, M., Sturm, M., Bertoglio, J., and Pallardy, M. (2001). Interleukin-2 inhibits glucocorticoid receptor transcriptional activity through a mechanism involving STAT5 (signal transducer and activator of transcription 5) but not AP-1. *Mol. Endocrinol. Baltim. Md.,* 15, 1062–1076.

Bons, J., Moreau, L., and Lefebvre, H. (2013). Adrenal disorders in human immunodeficiency virus (HIV) infected patients. *Ann. Endocrinol.*, 74, 508–514.

Bradley, W. G., Kraus, L. A., Good, R. A., and Day, N. K. (1995). Dehydroepiandrosterone inhibits replication of feline immunodeficiency virus in chronically infected cells. *Vet. Immunol. Immunopathol.*, 46, 159–168.

Brooke, S. M., and Sapolsky, R. M. (2000). The effects of steroid hormones in HIV-related neurotoxicity: a mini review. *Biol. Psychiatry,* 48, 881–893.

Brooke, S. M., and Sapolsky, R. M. (2002). Glucocorticoid exacerbation of gp120 neurotoxicity: role of microglia. *Exp. Neurol.,* 177, 151–158.

Brüggemeier, U., Rogge, L., Winnacker, E. L., and Beato, M. (1990). Nuclear factor I acts as a transcription factor on the MMTV promoter but competes with steroid hormone receptors for DNA binding. *EMBO J.*, 9, 2233–2239.

Bull, M. E., Vahlenkamp, T. W., Dow, J. L., Collisson, E. W., Winslow, B. J., Phadke, A. P., Tompkins, M. B., and Tompkins, W. A. F. (2004). Spontaneous T cell apoptosis in feline immunodeficiency virus (FIV)-infected cats is inhibited by IL2 and anti-B7.1 antibodies. *Vet. Immunol. Immunopathol.*, 99, 25–37.

Carmichael, K. P., Bienzle, D., and McDonnell, J. J. (2002). Feline leukemia virus-associated myelopathy in cats. *Vet. Pathol.*, 39, 536–545.

Chatterji, U., de Parseval, A., and Elder, J. H. (2002). Feline immunodeficiency virus OrfA is distinct from other lentivirus transactivators. *J. Virol.*, 76, 9624–9634.

Chittiprol, S., Shetty, K. T., Kumar, A. M., Bhimasenarao, R. S., Satishchandra, P., Subbakrishna, D. K., Desai, A., Ravi, V., Satish, K. S., Gonzalez, L., et al. (2007). HPA axis activity and neuropathogenesis in HIV-1 clade C infection. *Front. Biosci. J. Virtual Libr.*, 12, 1271–1277.

Chittiprol, S., Kumar, A. M., Shetty, K. T., Kumar, H. R., Satishchandra, P., Rao, R. S. B., Ravi, V., Desai, A., Subbakrishna, D. K., Philip, M., et al. (2009). HIV-1 clade C infection and progressive disruption in the relationship between cortisol, DHEAS and CD4 cell numbers: a two-year follow-up study. *Clin. Chim. Acta. Int. J. Clin. Chem.*, 409, 4–10.

Christeff, N., Gharakhanian, S., Thobie, N., Rozenbaum, W., and Nunez, E. A. (1992). Evidence for changes in adrenal and testicular steroids during HIV infection. *J. Acquir. Immune Defic. Syndr.*, 5, 841–846.

Christeff, N., Nunez, E. A., and Gougeon, M. L. (2000). Changes in cortisol/DHEA ratio in HIV-infected men are related to immunological and metabolic perturbations leading to malnutrition and lipodystrophy. *Ann. N. Y. Acad. Sci.*, 917, 962–970.

Christeff, N., De Truchis, P., Melchior, J.-C., Perronne, C., and Gougeon, M.-L. (2002a). Longitudinal evolution of HIV-1-associated lipodystrophy is correlated to serum cortisol:DHEA ratio and IFN-alpha. *Eur. J. Clin. Invest.*, 32, 775–784.

Christeff, N., De Truchis, P., Melchior, J.-C., Perronne, C., and Gougeon, M.-L. (2002b). Longitudinal evolution of HIV-1-associated lipodystrophy is correlated to serum cortisol:DHEA ratio and IFN-alpha. *Eur. J. Clin. Invest.*, 32, 775–784.

Clerici, M., Galli, M., Bosis, S., Gervasoni, C., Moroni, M., and Norbiato, G. (2000). Immunoendocrinologic abnormalities in human immunodeficiency virus infection. *Ann. N. Y. Acad. Sci.*, 917, 956–961.

Collado, V. M., Domenech, A., Miró, G., Martin, S., Escolar, E., and Gomez-Lucia, E. (2012). Epidemiological aspects and clinicopathological findings in cats naturally infected with feline leukemia virus (FeLV) and/or feline immunodeficiency virus (FIV). *Open J. Vet. Med.*, 2, 13–20.

Collazos, J., Ibarra, S., and Loureiro, M. (2004). Cortisol serum levels and their relationship to certain antiretroviral drugs. *Scand. J. Infect. Dis.,* 36, 480–482.

Costa, A., Nappi, R. E., Polatti, F., Poma, A., Grossman, A. B., and Nappi, G. (2000). Stimulating effect of HIV-1 coat protein gp120 on corticotropin-releasing hormone and arginine vasopressin in the rat hypothalamus: involvement of nitric oxide. *Exp. Neurol.,* 166, 376–384.

Diallo, K., Loemba, H., Oliveira, M., Mavoungou, D. D., and Wainberg, M. A. (2000). Inhibition of human immunodeficiency virus type-1 (HIV-1) replication by immunor (IM28), a new analog of dehydroepiandrosterone. *Nucleosides Nucleotides Nucleic Acids,* 19, 2019–2024.

Dimitrov, S., Lange, T., Fehm, H. L., and Born, J. (2004). A regulatory role of prolactin, growth hormone, and corticosteroids for human T-cell production of cytokines. *Brain. Behav. Immun.*, 18, 368–374.

De Parseval, A., and Elder, J. H. (1999). Demonstration that orf2 encodes the feline immunodeficiency virus transactivating (Tat) protein and characterization of a unique gene product with partial rev activity. *J. Virol.*, 73, 608–617.

Domenech, A., Tejerizo, G., Illera, J. C., and Gomez-Lucia, E. (2009). Effect of male steroid hormones on retroviral infections. *Curr. Top. Steroid Res.,* 6, 69–81.

Domenech, A., Gómez, N. V., and Gomez-Lucia, E. (2012). An update on the use of type I interferon for treating feline retrovirosis. In Felines. Behavior, Classification and Diseases (Animal Science, Issues and Professions), (New York: Nova Science Publishers, Inc), pp. 1–29.

Dudley, J. P., Mertz, J. A., Rajan, L., Lozano, M., and Broussard, D. R. (2002). What retroviruses teach us about the involvement of c-Myc in leukemias and lymphomas. *Leukemia,* 16, 1086–1098.

Dunham, S. P., and Graham, E. (2008). Retroviral infections of small animals. *Vet. Clin. North Am. Small Anim. Pract.,* 38, 879–901, ix.

Dunn, A. J., and Vickers, S. L. (1994). Neurochemical and neuroendocrine responses to Newcastle disease virus administration in mice. *Brain Res.*, 645, 103–112.

Fletcher, N. F., Brayden, D. J., Brankin, B., and Callanan, J. J. (2008). Feline immunodeficiency virus infection: a valuable model to study HIV-1 associated encephalitis. *Vet. Immunol. Immunopathol.*, 123, 134–137.

Fletcher, N. F., Bexiga, M. G., Brayden, D. J., Brankin, B., Willett, B. J., Hosie, M. J., Jacque, J.-M., and Callanan, J. J. (2009). Lymphocyte migration through the blood-brain barrier (BBB) in feline immunodeficiency virus infection is significantly influenced by the pre-existence of virus and tumour necrosis factor (TNF)-alpha within the central nervous system (CNS): studies using an in vitro feline BBB model. *Neuropathol. Appl. Neurobiol.*, 35, 592–602.

Fulkerson, W. J., and Tang, B. Y. (1979). Ultradian and circadian rhythms in the plasma concentration of cortisol in sheep. *J. Endocrinol.*, 81, 135–141.

Fulton, R., Plumb, M., Shield, L., and Neil, J. C. (1990). Structural diversity and nuclear protein binding sites in the long terminal repeats of feline leukemia virus. *J. Virol.*, 64, 1675–1682.

George, M. M., and Bhangoo, A. (2013). Human immune deficiency virus (HIV) infection and the hypothalamic pituitary adrenal axis. *Rev. Endocr. Metab. Disord.*, 14, 105–112.

Ghosh, D. (1992). Glucocorticoid receptor-binding site in the human immunodeficiency virus long terminal repeat. *J. Virol.*, 66, 586–590.

Ghosh, S.K., and Faller, D.V. (1999) Feline leukemia virus long terminal repeat activates collagenase IV gene expression through AP-1. *J. Virol.*, 73, 4931-40.

Gleich, S., and Hartmann, K. (2009). Hematology and serum biochemistry of feline immunodeficiency virus-infected and feline leukemia virus-infected cats. *J. Vet. Intern. Med. Am. Coll. Vet. Intern. Med.*, 23, 552–558.

Gómez, N. V., Castillo, V. A., Gisbert, M. A., Pisano, P., Mira, G., Fontanals, A., and Blatter, M. F. C. (2011). Immune-endocrine interactions in treated and untreated cats naturally infected with FIV. *Vet. Immunol. Immunopathol.*, 143, 332–337.

Gomez-Lucia, E., Tejerizo, G., and Domenech, A. (2007). Effect of steroid hormones on retroviruses. In Oncogenic Viruses Research Trends, (Hauppauge, NY: Nova Science), pp. 163–191.

Hapgood, J. P., and Tomasicchio, M. (2010). Modulation of HIV-1 virulence via the host glucocorticoid receptor: towards further understanding the molecular mechanisms of HIV-1 pathogenesis. *Arch. Virol.*, 155, 1009–1019.

Hartmann, K. (2011). Clinical aspects of feline immunodeficiency and feline leukemia virus infection. *Vet. Immunol. Immunopathol.*, 143, 190–201.

Hartmann, K. (2012). Clinical aspects of feline retroviruses: a review. *Viruses,* 4, 2684–2710.

Henderson, E., Yang, J. Y., and Schwartz, A. (1992). Dehydroepiandrosterone (DHEA) and synthetic DHEA analogs are modest inhibitors of HIV-1 IIIB replication. *AIDS Res. Hum. Retroviruses,* 8, 625–631.

Hofmann-Lehmann, R., Holznagel, E., and Lutz, H. (1998). Female cats have lower rates of apoptosis in peripheral blood lymphocytes than male cats: correlation with estradiol-17beta, but not with progesterone blood levels. *Vet. Immunol. Immunopathol.,* 65, 151–160.

Hofmann-Lehmann, R., Cattori, V., Tandon, R., Boretti, F. S., Meli, M. L., Riond, B., Pepin, A. C., Willi, B., Ossent, P., and Lutz, H. (2007). Vaccination against the feline leukaemia virus: outcome and response categories and long-term follow-up. *Vaccine*, 25, 5531–5539.

Ikeda, Y., Inoshima, Y., Kawaguchi, Y., Maeda, K., Kohmoto, M., Kai, C., Miyazawa, T., and Mikami, T. (1998). Protein-binding properties of the putative AP-1 and ATF sequences in the feline immunodeficiency virus long terminal repeat. *J. Gen. Virol.,* 79 (Pt 1), 95–99.

Inoshima, Y., Kohmoto, M., Ikeda, Y., Yamada, H., Kawaguchi, Y., Tomonaga, K., Miyazawa, T., Kai, C., Umemura, T., and Mikami, T. (1996). Roles of the auxiliary genes and AP-1 binding site in the long terminal repeat of feline immunodeficiency virus in the early stage of infection in cats. *J. Virol.*, 70, 8518–8526.

Jarrett, O. (2001). Feline leukaemia virus neutralising antibodies. *Vet. Rec.,* 149, 632.

Johnston, J. B., Silva, C., and Power, C. (2002). Envelope gene-mediated neurovirulence in feline immunodeficiency virus infection: induction of matrix metalloproteinases and neuronal injury. *J. Virol., 76*, 2622–2633.

Kino, T., Kopp, J. B., and Chrousos, G. P. (2000). Glucocorticoids suppress human immunodeficiency virus type-1 long terminal repeat activity in a cell type-specific, glucocorticoid receptor-mediated fashion: direct protective effects at variance with clinical phenomenology. *J. Steroid Biochem. Mol. Biol.*, 75, 283–290.

Kinter, A. L., Biswas, P., Alfano, M., Justement, J. S., Mantelli, B., Rizzi, C., Gatti, A. R., Vicenzi, E., Bressler, P., and Poli, G. (2001). Interleukin-6 and glucocorticoids synergistically induce human immunodeficiency virus type-1 expression in chronically infected U1 cells by a long terminal repeat independent post-transcriptional mechanism. *Mol. Med. Camb. Mass,* 7, 668–678.

Koirala, T. R., Sharma, S., Morikawa, S., and Ishida, T. (2000). Expression of CXCR4 in the brain of feline immunodeficiency virus infected cat. *Indian J. Pathol. Microbiol.,* 43, 285–290.

Kumar, M., Kumar, A. M., Waldrop, D., Antoni, M. H., Schneiderman, N., and Eisdorfer, C. (2002). The HPA axis in HIV-1 infection. *J. Acquir. Immune Defic. Syndr.*, 1999 31, Suppl. 2, S89–93.

Kurata, S. i, and Yamamoto, N. (1999). Glucocorticoid can reduce the transcriptional activation of HIV-1 promoter through the reduction of active NF-kappaB. *J. Cell. Biochem.,* 76, 13–19.

Lan, N. C., Karin, M., Nguyen, T., Weisz, A., Birnbaum, M. J., Eberhardt, N. L., and Baxter, J. D. (1984). Mechanisms of glucocorticoid hormone action. *J. Steroid Biochem.,* 20, 77–88.

Laudat, A., Blum, L., Guéchot, J., Picard, O., Cabane, J., Imbert, J. C., and Giboudeau, J. (1995). Changes in systemic gonadal and adrenal steroids in asymptomatic human immunodeficiency virus-infected men: relationship with the CD4 cell counts. *Eur. J. Endocrinol. Eur. Fed. Endocr. Soc.,* 133, 418–424.

Lawrence, C. E., Callanan, J. J., Willett, B. J., and Jarrett, O. (1995). Cytokine production by cats infected with feline immunodeficiency virus: a longitudinal study. *Immunology,* 85, 568–574.

Lawson, M. H., and Hosie, M. J. (2001). Follow up of feline immunodeficiency virus-infected cats. *Vet. Rec.,* 148, 449–450.

Levy, J. K., Liang, Y., Ritchey, J. W., Davidson, M. G., Tompkins, W. A., and Tompkins, M. B. (2004). Failure of FIV-infected cats to control Toxoplasma gondii correlates with reduced IL2, IL6, and IL12 and elevated IL10 expression by lymph node T cells. *Vet. Immunol. Immunopathol.*, 98, 101–111.

Lin, D. S., Bowman, D. D., and Jacobson, R. H. (1992). Immunological changes in cats with concurrent Toxoplasma gondii and feline immunodeficiency virus infections. *J. Clin. Microbiol.*, 30, 17–24.

Linenberger, M. L., and Deng, T. (1999). The effects of feline retroviruses on cytokine expression. *Vet. Immunol. Immunopathol.*, 72, 343–368.

Lu, W., Salerno-Goncalves, R., Yuan, J., Sylvie, D., Han, D. S., and Andrieu, J. M. (1995). Glucocorticoids rescue CD4+ T lymphocytes from activation-induced apoptosis triggered by HIV-1: implications for pathogenesis and therapy. *AIDS Lond. Engl.*, 9, 35–42.

Maingat, F. G., Polyak, M. J., Paul, A. M., Vivithanaporn, P., Noorbakhsh, F., Ahboucha, S., Baker, G. B., Pearson, K., and Power, C. (2012). Neurosteroid-mediated regulation of brain innate immunity in HIV/AIDS: DHEA-S suppresses neurovirulence. *FASEB J.*

Majors, J., and Varmus, H. E. (1983). A small region of the mouse mammary tumor virus long terminal repeat confers glucocorticoid hormone regulation on a linked heterologous gene. *Proc. Natl. Acad. Sci. U A,* 80, 5866–5870.

Marozsan, A. J., Fraundorf, E., Abraha, A., Baird, H., Moore, D., Troyer, R., Nankja, I., and Arts, E. J. (2004). Relationships between infectious titer, capsid protein levels, and reverse transcriptase activities of diverse human immunodeficiency virus type 1 isolates. *J. Virol.,* 78, 11130–11141.

Martin, M. E., Benassayag, C., Amiel, C., Canton, P., and Nunez, E. A. (1992). Alterations in the concentrations and binding properties of sex steroid binding protein and corticosteroid-binding globulin in HIV+patients. *J. Endocrinol. Invest.,* 15, 597–603.

Martin, P. A., and Crump, M. H. (2003). The adrenal gland. In McDonalds's Veterinary Endocrinology and Reproduction (5th Ed.), (Ames, Iowa: Iowa State Press),.

Mattsson, C., and Olsson, T. (2007). Estrogens and glucocorticoid hormones in adipose tissue metabolism. *Curr. Med. Chem.*, 14, 2918–2924.

McGrath, C. M. (1971). Replication of mammary tumor virus in tumor cell cultures: dependence on hormone-induced cellular organization. *J. Natl. Cancer Inst.,* 47, 455–467.

Mermod, N., Williams, T. J., and Tjian, R. (1988). Enhancer binding factors AP-4 and AP-1 act in concert to activate SV40 late transcription in vitro. *Nature,* 332, 557–561.

Mesbah, S., and Brudieux, R. (1982). Diurnal variation of plasma concentrations of cortisol, aldosterone and electrolytes in the ram. *Horm. Metab. Res. Horm. Stoffwechselforschung Horm. Métabolisme,* 14, 320–323.

Miksicek, R., Heber, A., Schmid, W., Danesch, U., Posseckert, G., Beato, M., and Schütz, G. (1986). Glucocorticoid responsiveness of the transcriptional enhancer of Moloney murine sarcoma virus. *Cell*, 46, 283–290.

Mirani, M., Elenkov, I., Volpi, S., Hiroi, N., Chrousos, G. P., and Kino, T. (2002). HIV-1 protein Vpr suppresses IL-12 production from human monocytes by enhancing glucocorticoid action: potential implications of Vpr coactivator activity for the innate and cellular immunity deficits observed in HIV-1 infection. *J. Immunol. Baltim. Md.,* 1950 169, 6361–6368.

Miró, G., Doménech, A., Escolar, E., Collado, V. M., Tejerizo, G., De Las Heras, A., and Gómez-Lucía, E. (2007). Plasma electrophoretogram in feline immunodeficiency virus (FIV) and/or feline leukaemia virus (FeLV) infections. *J. Vet. Med. A Physiol. Pathol. Clin. Med.,* 54, 203–209.

Mitra, D., Sikder, S. K., and Laurence, J. (1995). Role of glucocorticoid receptor binding sites in the human immunodeficiency virus type 1 long terminal repeat in steroid-mediated suppression of HIV gene expression. *Virology,* 214, 512–521.

Miyazawa, T., Kohmoto, M., Kawaguchi, Y., Tomonaga, K., Toyosaki, T., Ikuta, K., Adachi, A., and Mikami, T. (1993). The AP-1 binding site in the feline immunodeficiency virus long terminal repeat is not required for virus replication in feline T lymphocytes. *J. Gen. Virol.*, 74 *(Pt 8)*, 1573–1580.

Morrison, H. L., Soni, B., and Lenz, J. (1995). Long terminal repeat enhancer core sequences in proviruses adjacent to c-myc in T-cell lymphomas induced by a murine retrovirus. *J. Virol.,* 69, 446–455.

Muller, C., Hennebert, O., and Morfin, R. (2006). The native anti-glucocorticoid paradigm. *J. Steroid Biochem. Mol. Biol.*, 100, 95–105.

Murphy, B., Hillman, C., and McDonnel, S. (2014). Peripheral immunophenotype and viral promoter variants during the asymptomatic phase of feline immunodeficiency virus infection. *Virus Res.*, 179, 34–43.

Nair, M., Mahajan, S., Hou, J., Sweet, A. M., and Schwartz, S. A. (2000). The stress hormone, cortisol, synergizes with HIV-1 gp-120 to induce apoptosis of normal human peripheral blood mononuclear cells. *Cell. Mol. Biol. Noisy--Gd. Fr.*, 46, 1227–1238.

Niermann, G. L., and Buehring, G. C. (1997). Hormone regulation of bovine leukemia virus via the long terminal repeat. *Virology,* 239, 249–258.

Nishigaki, K., Endo, Y., Matsumoto, Y., Watari, T., Goitsuka, R., Tsujimoto, H., and Hasegata, A. (1997). Regulation of gene expression directed by the long terminal repeats of feline leukemia viruses. *Leukemia,* 11 Suppl. 3, 189–192.

Norbiato, G., Trifirò, G., Galli, M., Gervasoni, C., and Clerici, M. (2000). Fat redistribution in HIV-infected patients. A new hormonal-immune disorder? *Ann. N. Y. Acad. Sci.,* 917, 951–955.

Payvar, F., DeFranco, D., Firestone, G. L., Edgar, B., Wrange, Ö., Okret, S., Gustafsson, J.-Å., and Yamamoto, K. R. (1983). Sequence-specific binding of glucocorticoid receptor to MTV DNA at sites within and upstream of the transcribed region. *Cell*, 35, 381–392.

Pedersen, N. C., North, T. W., Rigg, R., Reading, C., Higgins, J., Leutenegger, C., and Henderson, G. L. (2003). 16alpha-Bromo-epiandrosterone therapy modulates experimental feline immunodeficiency virus viremia: initial enhancement leading to long-term suppression. *Vet. Immunol. Immunopathol.,* 94, 133–148.

Persidsky, Y., Stins, M., Way, D., Witte, M. H., Weinand, M., Kim, K. S., Bock, P., Gendelman, H. E., and Fiala, M. (1997). A model for monocyte migration through the blood-brain barrier during HIV-1 encephalitis. *J. Immunol. Baltim. Md.,* 1950 158, 3499–3510.

Peterson, K. E., and Chesebro, B. (2006). Influence of proinflammatory cytokines and chemokines on the neuropathogenesis of oncornavirus and immunosuppressive lentivirus infections. *Curr. Top. Microbiol. Immunol.,* 303, 67–95.

Podell, M., March, P. A., Buck, W. R., and Mathes, L. E. (2000). The feline model of neuroAIDS: understanding the progression towards AIDS dementia. *J. Psychopharmacol. Oxf. Engl.,* 14, 205–213.

Poreba, E., Goździcka-Józefiak, A., and Kedzia, H. (1998). Study on interaction of proteins isolated from epithelial cervical tissue with glucocorticoid-response element of HPV16. *Eur. J. Gynaecol. Oncol.*, 19, 394–398.

Poretsky, L., Can, S., and Zumoff, B. (1995). Testicular dysfunction in human immunodeficiency virus-infected men. *Metabolism*, 44, 946–953.

Poretsky, L., Song, L., Brillon, D. J., Ferrando, S., Chiu, J., McElhiney, M., Ferenczi, A., Sison, C., Haller, I., and Rabkin, J. (2009). Metabolic and hormonal effects of oral DHEA in premenopausal women with HIV infection: a randomized, prospective, placebo-controlled pilot study. Horm. Metab. Res. Horm. Stoffwechselforschung Horm. *Métabolisme,* 41, 244–249.

Power, C., Zhang, K., and van Marle, G. (2004). Comparative neurovirulence in lentiviral infections: The roles of viral molecular diversity and select proteases. *J. Neurovirol.*, 10 Suppl. 1, 113–117.

Quinn, G., and Langford, G. (2001). The porcine endogenous retrovirus long terminal repeat contains a single nucleotide polymorphism that confers distinct differences in estrogen receptor binding affinity between PERV A and PERV B/C subtypes. *Virology,* 286, 83–90.

Raber, J., Toggas, S. M., Lee, S., Bloom, F. E., Epstein, C. J., and Mucke, L. (1996). Central nervous system expression of HIV-1 Gp120 activates the hypothalamic-pituitary-adrenal axis: evidence for involvement of NMDA receptors and nitric oxide synthase. *Virology,* 226, 362–373.

Rabkin, J. G., McElhiney, M. C., Rabkin, R., McGrath, P. J., and Ferrando, S. J. (2006). Placebo-controlled trial of dehydroepiandrosterone (DHEA) for treatment of nonmajor depression in patients with HIV/AIDS. *Am. J. Psychiatry,* 163, 59–66.

Ramakrishnan, C., and Robins, D. M. (1997). Steroid hormone responsiveness of a family of closely related mouse proviral elements. *Mamm. Genome Off. J. Int. Mamm. Genome Soc.,* 8, 811–817.

Ringold, G., Lasfargues, E. Y., Bishop, J. M., and Varmus, H. E. (1975). Production of mouse mammary tumor virus by cultured cells in the absence and presence of hormones: assay by molecular hybridization. *Virology,* 65, 135–147.

Robert-Tissot, C., Rüegger, V. L., Cattori, V., Meli, M. L., Riond, B., Gomes-Keller, M. A., Vögtlin, A., Wittig, B., Juhls, C., Hofmann-Lehmann, R., et al. (2011). The innate antiviral immune system of the cat: molecular tools for the measurement of its state of activation. *Vet. Immunol. Immunopathol.*, 143, 269–281.

Rojko, J. L., and Kociba, G. J. (1991). Pathogenesis of infection by the feline leukemia virus. *J. Am. Vet. Med. Assoc.,* 199, 1305–1310.

Rojko, J., Essex, M., and Trainin, Z. (1988). Feline leukemia/sarcoma viruses and immunodeficiency. *Adv. Vet. Sci. Comp. Med.,* 32, 57–96.

Rojko, J. L., Hoover, E. A., Mathes, L. E., Krakowka, S., and Olsen, R. G. (1979). Influence of adrenal corticosteroids on the susceptibility of cats to feline leukemia virus infection. *Cancer Res.*, 39, 3789–3791.

Rojko, J. L., Fulton, R. M., Rezanka, L. J., Williams, L. L., Copelan, E., Cheney, C. M., Reichel, G. S., Neil, J. C., Mathes, L. E., and Fisher, T. G. (1992). Lymphocytotoxic strains of feline leukemia virus induce apoptosis in feline T4-thymic lymphoma cells. *Lab. Investig. J. Tech. Methods Pathol.*, 66, 418–426.

Rojko, J. L., Hartke, J. R., Cheney, C. M., Phipps, A. J., and Neil, J. C. (1996). Cytopathic feline leukemia viruses cause apoptosis in hemolymphatic cells. *Prog. Mol. Subcell. Biol.*, 16, 13–43.

Rousseau, G. G. (1984). Control of gene expression by glucocorticoid hormones. *Biochem. J.*, 224, 1–12.

Russo, F. O., Patel, P. C., Ventura, A. M., and Pereira, C. A. (1999). HIV-1 long terminal repeat modulation by glucocorticoids in monocytic and lymphocytic cell lines. *Virus Res.*, 64, 87–94.

Ruzek, M. C., Miller, A. H., Opal, S. M., Pearce, B. D., and Biron, C. A. (1997). Characterization of early cytokine responses and an interleukin (IL)-6-dependent pathway of endogenous glucocorticoid induction during murine cytomegalovirus infection. *J. Exp. Med.*, 185, 1185–1192.

Ryan, G., Grimes, T., Brankin, B., Mabruk, M. J. E. M. F., Hosie, M. J., Jarrett, O., and Callanan, J. J. (2005). Neuropathology associated with feline immunodeficiency virus infection highlights prominent lymphocyte trafficking through both the blood-brain and blood-choroid plexus barriers. *J. Neurovirol.,* 11, 337–345.

Sarvaiya, P. J., Schwartz, J. R., Geng, C., and Vedeckis, W. V. (2012). c-Myb interacts with the glucocorticoid receptor and regulates its level in pre-B-acute lymphoblastic leukemia cells. *Mol. Cell. Endocrinol.,* 361, 124–132.

Schifitto, G., McDermott, M. P., Evans, T., Fitzgerald, T., Schwimmer, J., Demeter, L., and Kieburtz, K. (2000). Autonomic performance and dehydroepiandrosterone sulfate levels in HIV-1-infected individuals: relationship to TH1 and TH2 cytokine profile. *Arch. Neurol.*, 57, 1027–1032.

Silverman, M. N., Pearce, B. D., Biron, C. A., and Miller, A. H. (2005). Immune Modulation of the Hypothalamic-Pituitary-Adrenal (HPA) Axis during Viral Infection. *Viral Immunol.,* 18, 41–78.

Simonetta, G., Walker, D. W., and McMillen, I. C. (1991). Effect of feeding on the diurnal rhythm of plasma cortisol and adrenocorticotrophic hormone concentrations in the pregnant ewe and sheep fetus. *Exp. Physiol.,* 76, 219–229.

Slater, E. P., Posseckert, G., Chalepakis, G., Redeuihl, G., and Beato, M. (1989). Binding of steroid receptors to the HREs of mouse mammary tumor virus, chicken and xenopus vitellogenin and rabbit uteroglobin genes: correlation with induction. *J. Steroid Biochem.,* 34, 11–16.

Smith, E. M., Meyer, W. J., and Blalock, J. E. (1982). Virus-induced corticosterone in hypophysectomized mice: a possible lymphoid adrenal axis. *Science,* 218, 1311–1312.

Smoller, C. G., Pitelka, D. R., and Bern, H. A. (1961). Cytoplasmic inclusion bodies in cortisol-treated mammary tumors of C3H/Crgl mice. *J. Biophys. Biochem. Cytol.*, 9, 915–920.

Soudeyns, H., Geleziunas, R., Shyamala, G., Hiscott, J., and Wainberg, M. A. (1993). Identification of a novel glucocorticoid response element within the genome of the human immunodeficiency virus type 1. *Virology,* 194, 758–768.

Sprague, W. S., TerWee, J. A., and VandeWoude, S. (2010). Temporal association of large granular lymphocytosis, neutropenia, proviral load, and FasL mRNA in cats with acute feline immunodeficiency virus infection. *Vet. Immunol. Immunopathol.,* 134, 115–121.

Stella, J., Croney, C., and Buffington, T. (2013). Effects of stressors on the behavior and physiology of domestic cats. *Appl. Anim. Behav. Sci.,* 143, 157–163.

Stewart, T. A., Hollingshead, P. G., and Pitts, S. L. (1988). Multiple regulatory domains in the mouse mammary tumor virus long terminal repeat revealed by analysis of fusion genes in transgenic mice. *Mol. Cell. Biol.,* 8, 473–479.

Teichmann, J., Stephan, E., Lange, U., Discher, T., Federlin, K., Stracke, H., Lohmeyer, J., Graef, V., and Bretzel, R. G. (1998). Evaluation of serum and urinary estrogen levels in male patients with HIV-infection. *Eur. J. Med. Res.*, 3, 533–537.

Tejerizo, G., Domenech, A., Illera, J. C., Collado, V. M., and Gomez-Lucia, E. (2005). Effect of 17beta-estradiol and progesterone on the expression of FeLV in chronically infected cells. *Vet. Microbiol.,* 109, 191–199.

Tejerizo, G., Doménech, A., Illera, J.-C., Silván, G., and Gómez-Lucía, E. (2012). Altered plasma concentrations of sex hormones in cats infected by feline immunodeficiency virus or feline leukemia virus. *Domest. Anim. Endocrinol.*, 42, 113–120.

Teng, C. S. (1990). Induction of feline immunodeficiency syndrome by feline leukemia virus: pituitary and adrenocortical dysfunctions. *AIDS Lond. Engl.*, 4, 1219–1224.

Thompson, F. J., Elder, J., and Neil, J. C. (1994). Cis- and trans-regulation of feline immunodeficiency virus: identification of functional binding sites in the long terminal repeat. *J. Gen. Virol.*, 75 (Pt 3), 545–554.

Tompkins, M. B., Bull, M. E., Dow, J. L., Ball, J. M., Collisson, E. W., Winslow, B. J., Phadke, A. P., Vahlenkamp, T. W., and Tompkins, W. A. (2002). Feline immunodeficiency virus infection is characterized by B7+CTLA4+ T cell apoptosis. *J. Infect. Dis.,* 185, 1077–1093.

Tshikuka, J. G., Torres-Anjel, M. J., Blenden, D. C., and Elliott, S. C. (1992). The microepidemiology of wasting syndrome, a common link to diarrheal disease, cancer, rabies, animal models of AIDS, and HIV-AIDS YHAIDS). The feline leukemia virus and rabies virus models. *Ann. N. Y. Acad. Sci.,* 653, 274–296.

Vahlenkamp, T. W., de Ronde, A., Schuurman, N. N., van Vliet, A. L., van Drunen, J., Horzinek, M. C., and Egberink, H. F. (1999). Envelope gene sequences encoding variable regions 3 and 4 are involved in macrophage tropism of feline immunodeficiency virus. *J. Gen. Virol.,* 80 (Pt 10), 2639–2646.

Vanitharani, R., Mahalingam, S., Rafaeli, Y., Singh, S. P., Srinivasan, A., Weiner, D. B., and Ayyavoo, V. (2001). HIV-1 Vpr transactivates LTR-directed expression through sequences present within -278 to -176 and increases virus replication in vitro. *Virology,* 289, 334–342.

Villette, J. M., Bourin, P., Doinel, C., Mansour, I., Fiet, J., Boudou, P., Dreux, C., Roue, R., Debord, M., and Levi, F. (1990). Circadian variations in plasma levels of hypophyseal, adrenocortical and testicular hormones in men infected with human immunodeficiency virus. *J. Clin. Endocrinol. Metab.*, 70, 572–577.

Wang, S. W., and Teng, C. S. (1994). Induction of feline acquired immune deficiency syndrome by feline leukemia virus: immuno- and neuroendocrine dysfunctions. *Proc. Soc. Exp. Biol. Med. Soc. Exp. Biol. Med. N. Y. N,* 205, 332–339.

Webb, M. S., Miller, A. L., Johnson, B. H., Fofanov, Y., Li, T., Wood, T. G., and Thompson, E. B. (2003). Gene networks in glucocorticoid-evoked apoptosis of leukemic cells. *J. Steroid Biochem. Mol. Biol.*, 85, 183–193.

Yang, J. Y., Schwartz, A., and Henderson, E. E. (1993). Inhibition of HIV-1 latency reactivation by dehydroepiandrosterone (DHEA) and an analog of DHEA. *AIDS Res. Hum. Retroviruses,* 9, 747–754.

Yoffe, J. R. (1981). Effects of inflammatory agents on endothelial lysosomal fragility and their inhibition by anti-inflammatory drugs. *Br. J. Pharmacol.*, 72, 603–608.

Zapanti, E., Terzidis, K., and Chrousos, G. (2008). Dysfunction of the hypothalamic-pituitary-adrenal axis in HIV infection and disease. *Horm. Athens Greece,* 7, 205–216.

Zhou, J., and Cidlowski, J. A. (2005). The human glucocorticoid receptor: one gene, multiple proteins and diverse responses. *Steroids,* 70, 407–417.

Zhu, Q., and Dudley, J. P. (2002). CDP binding to multiple sites in the mouse mammary tumor virus long terminal repeat suppresses basal and glucocorticoid-induced transcription. *J. Virol.*, 76, 2168–2179.

In: Felines
Editor: Colleen Kevins
ISBN: 978-1-63463-550-9

Chapter 2

NEW APPROACHES FOR HORMONAL CONTRACEPTION IN FEMALE CATS

Paulo Borges[1], Alain Fontbonne[1] and Rita Payan-Carreira[2]
[1]CERCA, ENVA. 7 avenue du Général de Gaulle, Maisons Alfort, France
[2]CECAV [Animal and Veterinary Sciences Research Centre] – Universidade de Trás-os-Montes e Alto Douro, Vila Real, Portugal

ABSTRACT

Though extensively used in the control of reproduction in domestic cats and in feral cat populations, medical contraception still raises concerns to the veterinary and the owners on respect to its safety and its efficiency. These concerns endorse, nowadays, the research in the development of new alternatives for effective, reversible and safe contraceptive methods for felids.

Hormonal contraceptives are intended for example, to master, in a reversible way, the reproductive cycle in genetically valuable cats, which presumes that they would be active for short periods of time and ought to safeguard the animal fertility.

However, hormonal contraceptives are also used worldwide to control the reproductive activity in either domestic or feral cats, for long-term treatments, because of a pretence short-term economical interest. Progestins are the most frequently used hormonal contraceptive in cats.

They are quite easy to obtain in some areas of the globe and relatively cheap; they have diverse drug presentations, which allow its use independently of the veterinary assistance, and are effective in preventing pregnancy. Still some undesirable side effects on health are attributed to progestins when used in long-term schedules or in older animals.

In the past decade, several new approaches to manage cats' reproduction were proposed to avoid the use of progestins. Cats have a very distinctive reproductive function compared to dogs. Based on their particularities (reviewed also in this chapter), alternative hormonal methods were proposed mainly targeting to abolish the GnRH secretion, thereby interfering with FSH and LH pulsatility and the endocrine control of gonads. Two different routes can achieve inhibition of the GnRH secretion: controlling directly the GnRH secretion, by the administration of a potent GnRH agonist, for example, or indirectly by manipulating melatonin concentrations (since cats are seasonal breeders), thus mimetizing a lengthened non-reproductive season. Some of these approaches are considered devoid of adverse effects on the reproductive tissues. Nevertheless some secondary effects have been found in practice.

This work intended to provide an overview of the current alternative methods regarding the classical approach, for the control of the reproductive cycle in domestic cats, along with the presentation of our experience considering the feline oestrous cycle. Based on our common practice, we would like to discuss the treatment schedules, the risks found during its clinical application and the future perspectives of using these molecules in contraception. In our opinion this information can be of outmost interest to students, clinicians or colonies' technicians, breeders and even to common pet owners.

1. Introduction

Cats, with a global population estimated at 600 million, are considered the most popular pets worldwide, and are adapted to all the environments and to different lifestyles. We can distinguish different types of cat populations, according to their living, which raise different concerns on respect to neutering or contraception (Levy and Crawford, 2004; Sparkes et al., 2013):

- The feral cats, born in the streets or born in the wild, born in the streets or born in the wild, which are totally dissociated from human contact;
- Stray abandoned cats, which retain and may even need human interaction;

- Street or community cats;
- Owned cats that lived outdoors for a considerable period of time;
- Household cats.

The prevalence and distribution of these different categories may differ among countries and is somehow influenced by cultural and social cues. The relative proportion of the first and second categories (feral and homeless cats) may bring important concerns on possible conflicts with the human population and on public health, as well as on their reflections on the ecology of particular wild species, traditionally preyed by felids (Levy and Crawford, 2004). In general, domestic cats present a highly efficient reproduction (Goericke-Pesch et al., 2014) that largely contributes to the stray feline overpopulation. Control of the reproductive activity in those particular populations has been in focus for long in an effort to control overpopulation. In this particular case, the target is a definitive contraception or sterilization of the animals, thus leading to the proposal of different forms of neutering. These are out of focus on the present chapter, where we envisaged presenting alternative methods for temporary contraception in cats.

Suspension of the regular reproductive activity is often envisaged worldwide; notwithstanding the reasons for such a request may deeply vary with the geographic region, the owners' plans or the available methods and its costs. Ideal methods for castration of feral populations, outdoor community owned animals or for responsible owners are usually clearly distinct from those available for the situations targeting a temporary suspension of the reproductive activity. Hormonal contraceptives cope with this goal and are frequently used to reversibly master the reproductive cycle in genetically valuable cats, which presumes that they would be active for short periods of time and ought to safeguard the animal fertility.

Though extensively used in the control of reproduction in domestic cats and in feral cat populations, medical contraception still raises concerns to the veterinary and the owners on respect to its safety and its efficiency. These concerns endorse, nowadays, the research in the development of new alternatives for effective, reversible, safe, practical and inexpensive contraceptive methods for domestic cats.

When selecting for a temporary contraceptive method, it is important to take into consideration the characteristics of the reproductive cycle in the species, because in many cases, they determine drugs and administration schedules. Consequently, after reviewing the reproductive cycles characteristics for domestic felids, currently available methods for hormonal contraception will be discussed on what concerns its efficiency, relative costs, side effects and on respect to reversion of the contraceptive effects.

2. The Estrous Cycle in the Domestic Cat

The onset of puberty in domestic cats (*Felis catus*, Linnaeus, 1758) occurs at an average of 8-10 months, but age at puberty can range from 4 months to 1 year depending on many factors (Stabenfeldt and Pedersen, 1991), such as the date of birth, genetics, nutrition, growth rate, the occurrence of illness, fur length (long-haired breeds reach puberty later than the short-haired) and the existence of positive social stimuli (presence of a male or cyclic females) (Tsutsui and Stabenfeldt, 1993; Fontbonne and Garnier, 1998).

Domestic cats are seasonally polyestrous, long-day breeders (Wildt et al., 1981). Anestrus occurs in short-length days, but the duration of seasonal anestrous greatly varies with the geographic location and the lifestyle. In the northern hemisphere, in regimes under natural daylight and temperature, the reproductive season may last from January to September, with a peak of activity in February and March (Tsutsui and Stabenfeldt, 1993; Fontbonne and Garnier, 1998; Feldman and Nelson, 2004). Household animals, maintained with fourteen hours of light and moderate environmental temperatures will maintain regular estrous cycles while anestrus may be minimal or non-existent (Tsutsui and Stabenfeldt, 1993; Johnston et al.1996). A decrease in the daily light to 8h or 10h suppresses the reproductive activity in cats, particularly if no social stimuli exist (Leyva et al., 1989; Fontbonne and Garnier, 1998).

Cats resume the estrous cycle quite early following parturition. In general, the first postpartum estrus may begin 10 days after weaning (Tsutsui and Stabenfeldt, 1993). It is currently believed that the litter number or the degree of the nipple stimulation during lactation may have a major effect on the suppression of the hypothalamus-pituitary axis that controls reproduction. But if presenting good body condition and adequate photoperiod, in the presence of a male, a discrete estrus may occur during weaning and may lead to pregnancy.

Cats present one distinctive particularity on their estrus cycle compared to dogs and other domestic animals: felids are reflex ovulators, i.e. ovulation is not spontaneous but triggered by mating. Receptors in the vagina, stimulated during the coitus, determine the releasing of LH within 5 min to 2 hours. The resulting LH peak will activate the ovulation cascade. Repeated matings are needed to ensure a consistent stimulation of LH surge (Tsutsui and

Stabenfeldt, 1993; Goericke-Pesch, 2010). Also, minimal estrogen priming is necessary to ensure a consistent LH surge and ovulation. Ovulation usually occurs 24-36h after copulation (Tsutsui and Stabenfeldt, 1993). Nevertheless, in some cases 25-30%), spontaneous ovulations have been observed in female cats (Gudemuth et al., 1997), that are more frequently described in animals living in larger groups, possibly in association to visual and pheromone stimuli (Gudemuth et al., 1997; Goericke-Pesch, 2010). Spontaneous ovulations are more frequent in young and older queens.

As a consequence of being a reflex ovulator species, cats may present two sorts of oestrous cycles: the anovulatory, if no ovulation ensues, or the ovulatory estrous cycle, when mating or spontaneous ovulation occurs. In the first situation, the cycle is characterized by successive follicular stages at 2 - 3 weeks interval and the inexistence of a luteal stage (Tsutsui and Stabenfeldt, 1993); while progesterone remains in basal values, consecutive follicular stages are separated by only a short non-follicular phase corresponding to the period of follicular atresia (Feldman & Nelson, 2004; Stornelli, 2007). For the non-ovulatory cycle, the interestrous interval (the period between two consecutive estrus) lasts an average of 9±7.6 days, ranging more frequently between 14 to 19 days (Stornelli, 2007). In cats, sexual behaviour corresponds mainly to estrus, although altered sexual behaviour may be seen 1-2 days before estrus and therefore this stage is named proestrus (Tsutsui and Stabenfeldt, 1993). Estrus lasts around 5 to 6 days, though in some females it may elongate up to 16 - 20 days (Fontbonne and Garnier, 1998).

In the case of ovulatory cycles, an alternancy of follicular and luteal stages is observed, although in cats the length of the luteal stage varies whether the female gets pregnant or not. The follicular phase (proestrus and estrus) is equally lengthened in ovulatory and anovulatory cycle. In contrast, the luteal stage is variable in the domestic cat: if the female achieves a pregnancy, the blood progesterone levels peak by day 21, and afterwards are maintained elevated up to days 52 to 74 days, due to the contribution of the placenta (Scott, 1970, cited by Fontbonne and Garnier, 1998). In the case where the female achieves spontaneous ovulation or does not get pregnant after mating (the later often named – erroneously – as pseudopregnancy; Fontbonne and Garnier, 1998), similar amounts of progesterone are produced by the corpora lutea, peaking also around day 21; afterwards, due to the absence of a pregnancy-associated stimulus the progesterone values drop more dramatically until they reach basal levels by 35 to 40 days post-ovulation (Verhage et al., 1976; Fontbonne and Garnier, 1998). Consequently, the interestrous interval is shorter if no mating occurs as estrus arise in 7 to 10 days after progesterone fall to basal values (corresponding to 45 to 50 days) comparing to the cases when the female conceives, where it takes 65 days to parturition in average (Verhage et al., 1976; Fontbonne and Garnier, 1998).

3. Non-Surgical Contraception in Cats

The pharmacological or chemical control of feline fertility may be achieved through sterilization, which definitively impairs animal reproduction, or by contraception, defined as a reversible method of blocking fertility (Massei and Miller, 2013) for a variable period, regarding the contraceptive method adopted. Pregnancy termination is not included on the contraception concept.

The need to control feline sexual activity has been traditionally endorsed through the administration of exogenous natural or synthetic progesterone molecules, either *per os* or systemically. By using this approach, the female is kept under a prolonged "artificial" luteal stage. However, other methods were recently tested in cats in an attempt to avoid the side effects of long-term progestagen administration, including the manipulation of GnRH secretion and the induction of anestrus based on the pharmacological control of the photoperiod.

In domestic cats, contraception is more widely used in females than in males. One possible explanation may be the desire to prevent estrus, thus reducing the occurrence of undesired pregnancies. Often, cat owners also whish to avoid surgical procedures, due either to financial constraints or to avoid some detrimental effects of a surgical castration. According to animal welfare legislation and ethical principles existing in some regions the need for non-surgical approach to domestic animals contraception is becoming a reality (Goericke-Pesch, 2010).

Pharmacologic methods of contraception and sterilization need to be safe, reliable, and reversible, and its use (schedules or doses) should be adjusted to the species´ physiology. Moreover, when opting for a specific contraceptive method, the veterinary practitioner need to consider the cat owner wishes, along with the expected benefits and the potential risks of the available methods. This procedure should be thoroughly discussed with the owner, having whenever needed an informed consent signed. It would be also important to judge the ability of the owner *vs.* the cat lifestyle to respect the adequate administration schedule, in order to minimize the side effects and to cope with the expected efficiency of the treatment.

Available contraceptive methods include hormonal treatments that act directly to block the reproductive hormones at the hypothalamus-pituitary-gonadal axis, such as progestins, or the GnRH agonists and melatonin; the two later methods have been proposed to avoid the side effects of long-term progestagen administration, by manipulation of GnRH secretion or the induction of anestrus based on the pharmacological control of photoperiod (Kutzler and Wood, 2007; Romagnoli and Sontas, 2010). The immuno-contraception, via vaccination against hormones or specific receptors of ovulated products oocyte, has been essayed in pets though its efficiency and the preservation of potential fertility has still to be proven (Kutzler and Wood, 2007; Romagnoli and Sontas, 2010; Goericke-Pesch, 2010). Additional methods investigated for mechanical disruption of fertility, such as the intravaginal or intra-uterine devices proved to be unsuitable for pets (Faulkner, 1975; Romagnoli and Sontas, 2010).

This section presents an overview of fertility control agents commercially available for cats. Once more we would like to strengthen that medical contraception must be intended for temporary suspension of feline sexual activity, in particular if exogenous progestins are used.

3.1. Progestins

Progestins (synthetic analogues of progesterone, also named progestogens) have been traditionally used worldwide as an alternative method for estrus suppression or estrus postponement in cats.

By using this approach, the female is kept under a prolonged artificial luteal stage, which is supposed to induce a down-regulation of the GnRH pulsatility, therefore compromising the release of FSH and LH in a cyclic pattern, necessary to ovarian follicular development. Progestins also alter the motility of the tubular reproductive tract, consequently impairing gamete transport and modifying the receptivity of a potential embryo by alteration of the viscosity and composition of tubal and uterine milieu (Munson, 2006; Goericke-Pesch, 2010; Goericke-Pesch et al., 2014).

Several important side effects have been attributed to progestins. These effects are related to their action in different systems and they are often associated with the incidence of side effects after chronic administration or if the administration timing and doses are not followed adequately. The actions and side effects of exogenous progestins are summarized on table 1. The drug, the duration of treatment and the schedule of administration determine the incidence in time for the development of side effects. Thus, one should be careful in the choice of the contraceptive treatment for a particular female.

Table 1. Summary of the exogenous progestins actions and related side effects

Main action	Effect	Negative side effect
Anti-gonadotrophic	↙ GnRH pulsatility ↙ FSH and LH secretion Folliculogenesis suspension Suppression of ovarian cycle	Increased time to restore fertility
Gestational	↗ Secretion by endometrial glands ↙ Myometrial contractibity Closure of the cervix Proliferation of the tubulo-alveolar tissue in the mammary gland	Mucometra and pyometra Mammary fibroepithelial hyperplasia Mammary neoplasia
Anti-estrogenic	Impair the reproductive tract contractibility and fluid movement, compromising gamete motility	Empowers the gestational effects
	Potential depression of ACTH secretion and the adrenal function with ↙ of cortisol levels	Hair discoloration Epidermal atrophy and alopecia
Non reproductive effects	Insulin resistance ↗ Insulin concentrations and disturbed glucose tolerance	Hyperglycemia and glycosuria *Diabetes mellitus*
	↗ Secretion of GH and IGF-I	Acromegaly Also favours development of diabetes

Main action	Effect	Negative side effect
	↗ Fat deposition due to stimulation of lipase ↙ Concentration of blood high density lipoproteins	Increased appetite and weight gain
	↙ Kidneys sodium retention due to ↙ aldosterone activity	
	Slight increase in the corporal temperature (thermogenic action)	
Other effects	Behavioural	Increase appetite and polyuria/polydipsia Increased weight ↙ overall activity
	In the site of injection	*Calcinosis circumscripta*

Administration of progestins is contraindicated in immature, non-pubertal females and in females presenting clinical evidences of hepatic, uterine, mammary or metabolic disease, which might be exacerbated by this contraceptive treatment (Romagnoli and Concannon, 2003; Goericke-Pesch, 2010). It is also important to discard an unaware pregnancy because the administration of progestogens during pregnancy might compromise pregnancy outcome and impair the normal onset of parturition (Romagnoli and Concannon, 2003). Although the progestins might be (exceptionally) administered also in the first days of behavioural estrus, it is recommended to started the treatment in anestrus or in the interestrous interval (Romagnoli and Sontas, 2010). Otherwise, accrue risks of acute severe side effects exist, in particular, the incidence of pyometra (Romagnoli and Concannon, 2003) and feline mammary adenomatous hyperplasia (Payan-Carreira, 2013). It is also important to remember that chronic treatments with progestins provoke changes in the animal body weight. Consequently, it is of utmost importance to avoid the use of fixed doses at the beginning and during progestin treatment in order to retard the development of associated side effects. Doses should always be adjusted to the female body weight (Goericke-Pesch, 2010; Romagnoli and Sontas, 2010). Also, one should be aware that exogenous progestins should not be administered for periods of more than 18 to 24 consecutive months (Kutzler and Wood, 2007; Romagnoli and Sontas, 2010) without a discontinuation period that should correspond from 2 to 3 months or 3 to 5 spontaneous cycles.

Through time, several products have been introduced in the market, with different antigonadotrophic, gestagenic and anti-estrogenic properties, which determine their potential to inducing negative side effects. Old generation drugs (such as medroxyprogesterone acetate or megestrol acetate) have usually stronger gestagenic action and consequently possess stronger negative side effects upon the mammary gland and the uterus, when chronically administered, than recent generation products (proligestone).

Medroxyprogesterone acetate (MPA) is widely used; it is sold in human and veterinary presentations either for oral (Perlutex® and Provera®, for example) or for parenteral administration (Supprestral® or Depo-Provera®, as examples). With a high antigonadotrophic action it possesses a long action; it also presents a high gestagenic action (Romagnoli and Concannon, 2003), meaning that it favors the negative effects associated with chronic progestagenic impregnation, in particular the mammary and uterine diseases and metabolic disturbances. This in fact determined that its use in small animals has not been approved in several countries. Because of its long action, MPA recommended dose for cats is 2.5mg/week/cat if oral formulations are used, or 2.0mg/cat at 5 months intervals in the case of systemic administration (Romagnoli and Sontas, 2010). The animals should be closely monitored for side effects, as this is the most aggressive progestin. Also it would be important to establish the treatment withdraw after 4 consecutive parenteral administrations or equivalent period if the oral presentation is used. Nevertheless, the use of MPA should be avoided in cats (Munson, 2006; Kutzler and Wood, 2007).

Megestrol acetate (MA) is a short-acting progestin, that is metabolised faster than MPA, thus with less negative side effects. MA is more fitted to temporary estrus suppression (Romagnoli and Concannon, 2003; Max et al., 2014). It is more commonly used as an oral formulation than as an injectable formulation. Possibly the most widely used compounds in feline practice are the presentations named Megecat® (by Vetoquinol) or Ovarid/Ovaban® (by Schering-Plough). Oral treatments with MA should start whilst in anestrus or during the interestrous interval, with a dose of 2.5 to 5 mg/cat/day for 3 to 5 days, followed by the same dose once a week (Munson, 2006). Romagnoli and

Sontas (2010) alternatively propose a dose of 5 mg/cat every 2 weeks, or half this dose per week. If the treatment is intend to start during behavioural estrus (it should be remembered that the risk of side effects is higher when treatments start during the follicular stage…) then the following regimen must be selected: 5 mg/cat/day until estrus stops (in general it takes 3-4 days), followed by a maintenance dose of 2.5 mg/cat/week or of 5 mg/cat every 2 weeks (Munson, 2006; Romagnoli and Sontas, 2010). Although safer than MPA, MA also presents some risks, mainly when the treatment schedule becomes irregular, due to the cat/owner lifestyle and also in older females treated *ad continuum* under constant (non weight-balanced) doses.

Delmadinone (DMA) and *Chlormadinone acetate* (CMA) are synthetic progestins with very limited diffusion in the global veterinary market. Similar to MPA, they are intended for prolonged estrus suppression or deferral and most frequently used as an injectable form. The recommended DMA (Tardak®) doses for cats are 2.5 to 5 mg/cat, sub-cutaneous, at 6 months intervals, starting in anestrus or in the interestrous interval. For estrus interruption it is recommended an initial treatment with 0.5 to 1.0mg/kg/day, sub-cutaneous, during 6 days, followed by the maintenance dose. Alternatively, it is possible to use one or two doses of 2.5 to 6.75mg/kg, 24h apart, followed by the maintenance dosage (Romagnoli and Sontas, 2010). CMA is presented in oral formulation, which can be applied to cats at weekly dosages of 2 to mg/cat (Jochle and Jochle, 1975; Tamada et al., 2003). To stop estrus, single oral doses of 5 mg of CMA at 24 hours intervals have been proposed, followed by the maintenance dose (Jochle and Jochle, 1975). Silastic implants with CMA in different dosages were experimented in cats; implants were left in place for one year. The minimal effective dose was 2.5mg/kg, and apparently it was devoid of short-term side effects on the uterus and mammary glands (Murakoshi et al., 2000). Limited information exists on these two products. Their actions are similar to those of MPA, thus similar side effects are expectable when used for long periods. CMA also possesses a stronger antiandrogen action that has been used in the aggressiveness control in different species. Return to estrus after treatment withdrawal is variable, but it is close to 8 months for DMA and up to 2 years for CMA (Romagnoli and Concannon, 2003).

Melengestrol acetate (MGA) is the most widely used contraceptive in zoo felids (Jewgenow et al., 2006), but it is seldom used in the domestic cat. Used as an implant, important side effects in uterus and mammary gland have been described in wild species (Munson, 2006).

Proligestone (PRG) is a new generation synthetic progestin with a larger antigonadotrophic action but weaker gestational and antiestrogenic effects compared to MPA and MA (Kutzler and Wood, 2007; Max et al., 2014). Recommended doses for PRG (Delvosteron®/Covinan®, Intervet) in cats is 10mg/kg, subcutaneously, repeated sequentially after 3 and 4 months, and thereafter at 5 months intervals (Romagnoli and Sontas, 2010); treatment should start during interestrous interval or anestrus. Return to spontaneous estrus is expected in 8 months after treatment withdraw. However, this regimen, adapted from the one prescribed in dogs, raises many questions if the reproductive cycle of the domestic cat is taken into consideration. PLG can be used at the dosage of 30mg/cat (Findik et al., 1999), every 6 months, starting in anestrus or during the interestrous interval. If treatment starts during diestrus, resumption of spontaneous estrus may occur around 4-5 months after administration (Findik et al., 1999), thus it may be advisable to measure progesterone levels one week after estrus to adjust the schedule of the first two administrations. PRG is considered a safer drug than older progestins, and reported to have minimal side effects (Kutzler and Wood, 2007; Goericke-Pesch et al., 2014; Max et al., 2014).

3.2. Androgens

Along with progestins, androgens (either natural or synthetic) have the ability to down-regulate the hypothalamus-pituitary-gonadal function and therefore might be used for estrus prevention (Munson, 2006). However, the anabolic effects and the associated virilisation of treated animals are important issues concerning androgen administration. Signs of virilisation, including clitoral hypertrophy, urine-spraying and thickness of the cervical skin, tend to persist after treatment withdrawal (Kutzler and Wood, 2007). Additional side effects described for androgen contraceptive treatments include vaginitis and urinary incontinence (Romagnoli and Sontas, 2010). Mibolerone, a synthetic androgen available for dogs, is not advisable for use in cats (Max et al., 2014), because in this species the minimal effective dose (50μg/day) is too close to the toxic dose and induces a short-term hepatic dysfunction (Kutzler and Wood, 2007).

3.3. GnRH Agonists

Agonists of GnRH target to suppress GnRH pulsatility and consequently that of LH and FSH; indirectly, these compounds abolish the secretion of sexual steroids. Briefly, they set the animal (male or female) into a pre-pubertal stage again, removing the sex steroid influences over gonads or behaviour. Therefore, they would greatly contribute to a reduction in the risks of uterine and mammary diseases usually associated to progesterone and are helpful in controlling undesirable sexual behaviour such as heat, urine spraying and aggressiveness. Nowadays, their main constraint is the price, which is not competitive towards that of progestins.

Sustained exposition to a GnRH agonist would override endogenous pulsatile GnRH due to a combined action at the levels of GnRH receptor that include receptor down-regulation, internalization and signal uncoupling (Kutzler and Wood, 2007). GnRH agonists are available as short or long-term contraceptives (Ackermann et al., 2012; Maenhoudt et al., 2012; Risso et al., 2012; Toydemir et al., 2012) and have the advantage that they may be used without apparent side effects to postpone puberty (Goericke-Pesch et al., 2013a; Schäfer-Somi et al., 2014).

Several synthetic molecules have been tried, including buserelin (50 μg, single administration) and azagly-nafarelin (Gonazon® implant), but the most studied commercial sources of GnRH agonist are deslorelin acetate implants (Suprelorin®, Virbac) and leuprolide acetate (Lupron Depot®, Abbott). Limited availability is a main constrain to a more widespread use, since these drugs have not been associated with significant adverse health effects in the cat (Munson, 2006). Deslorelin acetate (Suprelorin) is presented as 4.7 mg or 9.4 mg implants.

The most important undesirable effect of GnRH agonists for contraception is the flare-up effect. This effect is associated to an initial rise in FSH and LH concentrations that precedes the down regulation of GnRH secretion, and in the female it is responsible for the expression of a fertile estrus when administered out of a luteal phase (Ackermann et al., 2012; Goericke-Pesch et al., 2013a). This flare-up effect is poorly described, but it seems to present some individual variation. Nevertheless, this is not observed when the treatment starts in early diestrus, when progesterone concentrations are elevated. It seems that induced estrus is similarly lengthened compared to spontaneous estrus (Ackermann et al., 2012) The treatment of an unknown pregnant female cat did not interfere with the pregnancy course and allowed normal parturition, but it was accompanied by agalactia and failure of maternal behaviour expression (Goericke-Pesch et al., 2013b).

Implants are injected subcutaneously at the interscapular or the umbilical area (easier to remove if needed). The need for tranquilization of the animal remains to be proved, but it may depend essentially on the local of inoculation and on the cat temperament, being eventually advantageous to perform local anaesthesia. Changes may be observed at the place of inoculation (Toydemir et al., 2012): a small orifice remains at the implant site for 1-2 days; small capillary haemorrhages may occur, which are rapidly overcame; slight oedema can remain for 2-3 days, but there should be no signs of inflammation or infection. In a very small number of animals, very slight scratching lesions in the shaved areas have been observed. The implant remains detectable for long periods (up to 18 months; Toydemir et al., 2012), which allows its removal in short-term treatments (Ackermann et al., 2012).

Although treatment efficacy may vary in an individual basis, 4.7 mg implants proved to be effective to suppress the reproductive activity for 12 - 36 months (Romagnoli and Sontas, 2010; Goericke-Pesch et al., 2014). Time to resumption of spontaneous ovarian cycles depends on whether the implants are left in place or removed. Shorter treatments may be obtained if the implants are removed earlier. If removed after 2 months, spontaneous estrus cycle occurs in an average of 42 days (Ackermann et al., 2012). In a recent work, Goericke-Pesch and collaborators (2013a) obtained normal fertility rates after the end of a single implantation, resulting in the suppression of the reproductive activity for an average length of 650 days.

Ideally, to avoid estrus induction, treatments would start in diestrus. In one experiment (Toydemir et al., 2012) the use of a 9.4 mg implant in association with the administration of 3 doses of 5 mg megestrol acetate, PO (on the 14th day and at 12 hours before the implantation, and again on the 14th day after the implant inoculation) avoided the flare-up effect.

In proposed treatments to postpone puberty, a 4.7mg implant should be applied when the female reaches 50% of her mature body weight, corresponding to a period between 4 to 6 months of age; however, the success may vary individually and several doses may be needed (Risso et al., 2012; Schäfer-Somi et al., 2014). In a recent trial, Carranza et al. (2014) obtained a clear delay in puberty (around 15 months in female cats) by inoculating newborn kittens within 24 h after birth with a 1.6 mg deslorelin implant. Fertility was maintained in 11 out of the 16 females tested. However, this method evidenced a wide range of efficacy suggestive of different individual idiosyncratic factors.

Disturbed body development was not recorded in any of the studies on puberty postponement using deslorelin (Schäfer-Somi et al., 2014). Moreover, removal of the implant or the interruption of consecutive treatments shortens the contraceptive effect and allow the female to resume cyclic ovarian activity up, if it is removed before the end of the releasing action.

3.4. GnRH Antagonists

Antagonists of GnRH bind to GnRH receptors blocking its action, thus compromising the function of the hypothalamus-pituitary-gonadal axis. Long-term effects also include the down-regulation of GnRH receptors (Kutzler and Wood, 2007; Goericke-Pesch et al., 2014). Available GnRH antagonists tested in cats are Antide® and Acyclin®.

Using acycline, administered once at a dosage of 330 μg/kg, SC, to females cohabiting with a proven male, Risso et al. (2010) report that estrus was not interrupted in treated female cats, comparing to the control group animals; nevertheless, ovulation and subsequent pregnancy were impaired by treatment.

Antide® was also tested for suppression of ovarian activity in the domestic cat. A treatment with two 6 mg/kg injections given 15 days apart allowed prevention of spontaneous ovulation, but failed to induce ovarian down-regulation or coitus-induced ovulation (Pelican et al. 2005; Pelican et al. 2008); thereby, this class of drugs show a low efficiency as contraceptives in the cat, compared to other domestic carnivores species.

3.5. Melatonin

In the recent years, a new approach on temporary contraception has been explored for cats, taking advantage of the species seasonality and the fact that anestrous season occurs in winter, when melatonin levels peak. Melatonin implants were used to mime the endogenous mechanism controlling the onset of winter non-reproductive season and to induce an anestrous condition: elevated melatonin levels repress GnRH secretion and thereby decreases the secretion of LH and FSH. Consequently, the ovarian activity is suspended. In the first studies, oral melatonin regimens have been essayed (Graham et al., 2004; Faya et al., 2011). However, such regimens are impractical because of the need for a daily administration (the dose depending on the formulation) that will last for a variable period (in the experimental studies it varied from 35 days, up to 50 days or until estrus onset), allied to the fact that pills must be administered 2 to 3 hours before onset of darkness (which may be more difficult to establish among in-house animals that might be submitted to periods of artificial illumination at the end of the day).

A more reasonable approach recommends the application of a subcutaneous melatonin implant (Melovine® 18mg, CEVA Santé Animal) for temporary estrus suppression. Melatonin implants should be inoculated at the interscapular or the umbilical area, under the necessary aseptic conditions. Melatonin implants should be placed during the interestrous interval. When inoculated at this stage, anestrus is twice longer compared to the obtained with melatonin implantation during estrus (around 110 days *vs.* 60 days, respectively) (Gimenez et al., 2009; Faya et al., 2011).

Starting the melatonin treatment in periods outside the reproductive season (in anestrus or before puberty) did not prove to bring advantages (Gulyuz et al., 2009; Faya et al., 2011). One study, enrolling Turkish Van cats, tested the effects of melatonin implants placed during the anestrus season on the suspension of ovarian activity (Gulyuz et al., 2009). Implants were inoculated in mid December and removed by early April when the light cycle was of 13 hours. Treatment postponed the onset of the breeding season in females treated with melatonin in comparison to controls; however, it could not completely suspend ovarian activity once the daylight increased over a threshold of 13h of light (Gulyuz et al., 2009).

In prepubertal females, treatment with melatonin implants did not significantly postpone puberty, although females were slightly older (close to 40 days) when expressing estrus, compared to controls. Body weight at puberty was equal for treated and non-treated animals (Faya et al., 2011).

Little information is available on putative side effects of melatonin implants. Faya et al. (2011) refer the inexistence of uterine disease in treated animals, an information also advanced by Gimenez et al. (2009); however those were short-term studies that enrolled animals aged between 1 and 4 years of age. Nevertheless, it is not expectable to find evidences of side effects concerning diseases associated to sex steroids in healthy animals. Still, it would be of interest to assess its possible beneficial effects on the evolution and treatment of uterine and mammary diseases in older animals. In addition to its influences upon the sexual activity, melatonin also interferes with other body systems and endocrine mechanisms. Its actions over the metabolism, in particular on the weight gain and fat deposition, or on the thyroid function, the fur coat and skin are still missing, and may be of value for particular cat breeds.

3.6. Immune Contraception

Classical targets in immunocontraception include the GnRH and LH along with their corresponding receptors, for suspension of the cyclic activity, as well as the *zona pellucida* (ZP) proteins, in order to inhibit fertilization. Either approach shows unsatisfactory results till present.

Anti-GnRH vaccines (such as GonaCom®) induced suspension of ovarian activity for periods that varied from 5 months to 5 years with a single application. Moreover, time to conception is quite long (close to 40 months in average), which was associated with persistence of high GnRH antibody titers. Gender differences have been reported, with females being more sensitive to the vaccine effects (Levy et al., 2011).

Zona pellucida vaccines have been tested in cats, but their ability to achieve complete contraception is limited (Eade et al., 2009) when using specific antibodies for feline ZP while antibodies generated against porcine ZP were devoid of effect (Gorman et al., 2002). Another inconvenient is that the estrus cycle is not suspended, leaving the animal as susceptive to uterine and mammary diseases as any other intact female, while also expressing normal estrus behaviour (Eade et al., 2009).

A major side effect is the development of long-lasting granulomatous lesions at the place of inoculation (Munson et al., 2005; Levy et al., 2011). This issue is particularly important in cats, which is a species predisposed to the feline fibrosarcoma complex, a malignant neoplasia.

Conclusion

A variety of drugs are available for contraception in domestic cats. Most of advantages and inconveniences for each one have been discussed above. These should be carefully considered, along with the intended purpose of the treatment (short- or long-term treatments *vs.* sterilization), the schedule of administrations and the costs of the therapeutics, when presenting the owner the best option for a contraception approach for his/her female cat. Moreover, the contraception should be tailored for each individual female, and the owner capacity to cope with the selected regiment should be evaluated, as it strongly contributes to the success of the treatment. Age, reproductive status and the existence of a putative disease (independently of the system involved) should be taken into account, as they may influence the efficiency and the occurrence of side effects. Not all of the products meet the minimum safety requirements and it is the practitioner´s responsibility to warn and anticipate possible complications. In recent years, new products were tested for cats; although short-term studies demonstrated that they are safer than the traditional progestins used as contraceptives, long-term studies are needed to investigate their effects on the female's health, in particular under chronic administration.

References

Ackermann C. L.; Volpato R.; Destro F. C.; Trevisol E.; Sousa N. R.; Guaitolini C. R.; Derussi A. A.; Rascado T. S.; Lopes M. D., 2012: Ovarian activity reversibility after the use of deslorelin acetate as a short-term contraceptive in domestic queens. *Theriogenology,* 78 817-822.

Carranza A.; Faya M.; Merlo M. L.; Batista P.; Gobello C., 2014: Effect of GnRH analogs in postnatal domestic cats. *Theriogenology,* 82 138-143.

Eade J. A.; Roberston I. D.; James C. M., 2009b: Contraceptive potential of porcine and feline zona pellucida A, B and C subunits in domestic cats. *Reproduction,* 137 913-922.

Faulkner L. C., 1975: Contraceptive technology in controlled reproduction in pets. *American Journal of Public Health,* 65 77-78.

Faya M.; Carranza A.; Priotto M.; Graiff D.; Zurbriggen G.; Diaz J. D.; Gobello C., 2011: Long-term melatonin treatment prolongs interestrus, but does not delay puberty, in domestic cats. *Theriogenology,* 75 1750-1754.

Feldman E.C.; Nelson R.W., 2004: Feline Reproduction. *In: Canine and Feline Endocrinology and Reproduction. Saunders - Elsevier Health Sciences,* St. Louis, Missouri, USA, 1016 – 1045.

Findik M.; Maral N.; Aslan S., 1999: The use of proligestone, megestrol acetate and GnRH on queens with the aim of hormonal contraception. *Turkish Journal of Veterinary & Animal Sciences,* 23 455-459.

Fontbonne A.; Garnier F., 1998. Données récentes en physiologie et endocrinologie sexuelles dans l´espèce féline. *Le Point Veterinaire,* 29 1107-1112.

Gimenez F.; Stornelli M. C.; Tittarelli C. M.; Savignone C. A.; Dorna I. V.; de la Sota R. L.; Stornelli M. A., 2009: Suppression of estrus in cats with melatonin implants. *Theriogenology,* 72 493-499.

Goericke-Pesch S., 2010: Reproduction control in cats: new developments in non-surgical methods. *J Feline Med Surg,* 12 539-546.

Goericke-Pesch S.; Georgiev P.; Atanasov A.; Albouy M.; Navarro C.; Wehrend A., 2013a: Treatment of queens in estrus and after estrus with a GnRH-agonist implant containing 4.7 mg deslorelin; hormonal response, duration of efficacy, and reversibility. *Theriogenology,* 79 640-646.

Goericke-Pesch S.; Georgiev P.; Atanasov A.; Wehrend A., 2013b: Treatment with Suprelorin in a pregnant cat. *J Feline Med Surg,* 15 357-360.

Goericke-Pesch S.; Wehrend A.; Georgiev P., 2014: Suppression of fertility in adult cats. *Reprod Domest Anim,* 49 Suppl 2 33-40.

Gorman SP, Levy JK, Hampton AL, Collante WR, Harris AL, Brown RG. Evaluation of a porcine zona pellucida vaccine for the immunocontraception of domestic kittens (Felis catus). *Theriogenology.* 2002.

Graham L. H.; Swanson W. F.; Wildt D. E.; Brown J. L., 2004: Influence of oral melatonin on natural and gonadotropin-induced ovarian function in the domestic cat. *Theriogenology,* 61 1061-1076.

Gudermuth D. F.; Newton L Fau - Daels P.; Daels P Fau - Concannon P.; Concannon P., *Incidence of spontaneous ovulation in young, group-housed cats based on serum and faecal concentrations of progesterone.*

Gulyuz F.; Tasal I; Uslu B.A., 2009. Effects of Melatonin on the Onset of Ovarian Activity in Turkish Van Cats. *Journal of Animal and Veterinary Advances,* 8 2033-2037.

Jewgenow K.; Dehnhard M.; Hildebrandt T. B.; Göritz F., 2006: Contraception for population control in exotic carnivores. *Theriogenology,* 66 1525-1529.

Jöchle W.; Jöchle M., 1975: Reproductive and behavioral control in the male and female cat with progestins: long-term field observations in individual animals. *Theriogenology,* 3 179-185.

Johnston S. D.; Kustritz M. V.; Olson P. N., 2001: The Feline Estrous Cycle. Canine and Feline *Theriogenology.* Saunders - Elsevier, Philadelphia, USA, 396-405.

Kutzler M.; Wood A., 2006: Non-surgical methods of contraception and sterilization. *Theriogenology,* 66 514-525.

Levy J. K.; Crawford P. C., 2004: Humane strategies for controlling feral cat populations. *J Am Vet Med Assoc,* 225 1354-1360.

Levy J. K.; Friary J. A.; Miller L. A.; Tucker S. J.; Fagerstone K. A., 2011: Long-term fertility control in female cats with GonaCon™, a GnRH immunocontraceptive. *Theriogenology,* 76 1517-1525.

Leyva H; Madley T; Stabenfeldt GH, 1989. Effect of melatonin on photoperiod responses, ovarian secretion of oestrogen, and coital responses in the domestic cat. *J Reprod Fertil, Suppl.* 39 35-42.

Maenhoudt C.; Santos N. R.; Fontaine E.; Mir F.; Reynaud K.; Navarro C.; Fontbonne A., 2012: Results of GnRH agonist implants in oestrous induction and oestrous suppression in bitches and queens. *Reprod Domest Anim,* 47 Suppl 6 393-397.

Massei G.; Miller L. A., 2013: Nonsurgical fertility control for managing free-roaming dog populations: a review of products and criteria for field applications. *Theriogenology,* 80 829-838.

Max A.; Jurka P.; Dobrzy´nski A; Rijsselaere T., 2014. Non-surgical contraception in female dogs and cats. *Acta Sci. Pol., Zootechnica,* 13 3–18.

Munson L., 2006: Contraception in felids. *Theriogenology,* 66 126-134.

Munson L.; Harrenstien L. A.; Acton A. E.; Graham P. A.; Chassy L. M.; Kirkpatrick J. F., 2005: Immunologic responses and adverse reactions to Freund's-adjuvanted porcine zona pellucida immuno-contraceptives in domestic cats. *Vaccine,* 23 5646-5654.

Murakoshi M.; Tagawa M.; Ikeda R., 2000: Histopathological studies of subcutaneous implantation of chlormadinone acetate (CMA) for preventing estrus in queens. *Tokai J Exp Clin Med,* 25 7-10.

Payan-Carreira R., 2013 - Feline Mammary Fibroepithelial Hyperplasia: A Clinical Approach. *In:* Insights from Veterinary Medicine, Dr. Rita Payan Carreira (Ed.), ISBN: 978-953-51-1005-7, InTech, Available from: http://www.intechopen.com/books/insights-from-veterinary-medicine/ feline-mammary-fibroepithelial-hyperplasia-a-clinical-approach [accessed on june 23, 2014].

Pelican K. M.; Brown J. L.; Wildt D. E.; Ottinger M. A.; Howard J. G., 2005: Short term suppression of follicular recruitment and spontaneous ovulation in the cat using levonorgestrel versus a GnRH antagonist. *Gen Comp Endocrinol,* 144 110-121.

Pelican K. M.; Wildt D. E.; Ottinger M. A.; Howard J., 2008: Priming with progestin, but not GnRH antagonist, induces a consistent endocrine response to exogenous gonadotropins in induced and spontaneously ovulating cats. *Domest Anim Endocrinol,* 34 160-175.

Risso A.; Corrada Y.; Barbeito C.; Diaz J. D.; Gobello C., 2012: Long-term-release GnRH agonists postpone puberty in domestic cats. *Reprod Domest Anim,* 47 936-938.

Risso A.; Valiente C.; Corrada Y.; Romero G. G.; Blanco P. G.; de la Sota P. E.; Diaz J. D.; Gobello C., 2010: The GnRH antagonist acyline prevented ovulation, but did not affect ovarian follicular development or gestational corpora lutea in the domestic cat. *Theriogenology,* 73 984-987.

Romagnoli S., 2010: Reproduction control - new developments, old debates. *J Feline Med Surg,* 12 724.

Romagnoli S.; Concannon P.W., 2003. Clinical use of progestins in bitches and queens: a review. *Recent Advances in Small Animals Reproduction* 2003. available on-line at www.ivis.org. Document No. A1206.0903 [accessed on september 5, 2014].

Romagnoli S.; Sontas B.H., 2010. Prevention of breeding in the female. *In*: *BSAVA Manual of Canine and Feline Reproduction and Neonatology,* 2nd Edition, Gary England and Angelika von Heimendahl (Editors), British Small Animal Veterinary Association, Gloucester, UK, 23-33.

Schäfer-Somi S.; Kaya D.; Gültiken N.; Aslan S., 2014: Suppression of fertility in pre-pubertal dogs and cats. *Reprod Domest Anim,* 49 Suppl 2 21-27.

Sparkes A. H.; Bessant C.; Cope K.; Ellis S. L.; Finka L.; Halls V.; Hiestand K.; Horsford K.; Laurence C.; MacFarlaine I.; Neville P. F.; Stavisky J.; Yeates J.; ISFM, 2013: ISFM guidelines on population management and welfare of unowned domestic cats (Felis catus). *J Feline Med Surg,* 15 811-817.

Stabenfeldt G.H.; Pedersen N.C., 1991. Reproduction and reproductive disorders. *In*: *Feline Husbandry. Disease and management in the multiple-cat environment.* NC Pedersen (Editor), American Veterinary Publications, Goleta, California: 129-162.

Stewart R. A.; Pelican K. M.; Brown J. L.; Wildt D. E.; Ottinger M. A.; Howard J. G., 2010: Oral progestin induces rapid, reversible suppression of ovarian activity in the cat. *Gen Comp Endocrinol,* 166 409-416.

Stornelli M.A., 2007. Particularidades fisiológicas de la reproducción en felinos. *Rev Bras Reprod Anim, Belo Horizonte,* 31 71-76.

Tamada H.; Kawate N.; Inaba T.; Sawada T., 2003: Long-term prevention of estrus in the bitch and queen using chlormadinone acetate. *Can Vet J,* 44 416-417.

Toydemir T. S.; Kılıçarslan M. R.; Olgaç V., 2012: Effects of the GnRH analogue deslorelin implants on reproduction in female domestic cats. *Theriogenology,* 77 662-674.

Tsutsui T.; Stabenfeldt G. H., 1993: Biology of ovarian cycles, pregnancy and pseudopregnancy in the domestic cat. *J Reprod Fertil Suppl,* 47 29-35.

Verhage H. G.; Beamer N. B.; Brenner R. M., 1976: Plasma levels of estradiol and progesterone in the cat during polyestrus, pregnancy and pseudopregnancy. *Biol Reprod,* 14 579-585.

Wildt D. E.; Chan S. Y.; Seager S. W.; Chakraborty P. K., 1981: Ovarian activity, circulating hormones, and sexual behavior in the cat. I. Relationships during the coitus-induced luteal phase and the estrous period without mating. *Biol Reprod,* 25 15-28.

In: Felines
Editor: Colleen Kevins

ISBN: 978-1-63463-550-9

Chapter 3

FELINE IMMUNODEFICIENCY VIRUS INFECTION

Sheila de Oliveira Medeiros[1] and Julia Pierucci[2]
[1]Universidade Federal do Rio de Janeiro-UFRJ - Rio de Janeiro-RJ, Brazil
[2]Universidade Estadual Paulista - UNESP - Sao Paulo SP, Brazil

ABSTRACT

Feline Immunodeficiency Virus (FIV) is one of most common feline viral diseases, affecting wild and domestic cats worldwide. FIV belongs to the Retroviridae family, the most famous representative of which is Human Immunodeficiency Virus (HIV). The main mode of transmission is through bite wounds, but vertical transmission is also possible. Based on the mode of transmission, unneutered male outdoor cats are the highest-risk group. The infection is characterized by a long incubation period and a persistent infection, with development of acquired immune deficiency syndrome (AIDS), similar to HIV. In this stage the cat is susceptible to secondary and opportunistic infections. Infected cats may develop different clinical conditions, such as tumors and renal disease, but one of the most common manifestations is oral cavity disease. An FIV vaccine is available, but identification and isolation of infected cats is recommended as a preventive measure. FIV was isolated in 1986 in a colony of cats with opportunistic infections. Since then, relatively little research has been done on some aspects of the infection, like chronic or terminal stages of the disease, and mainly with respect to antiviral treatment.

The purpose of this chapter is to update, through literature review, some aspects of clinical, epidemiological, diagnostics and treatments of FIV infection in the domestic cat.

INTRODUCTION

Retroviruses were described for the first time in animals and became important models for cellular and molecular studies, contributing to the discovery of oncogenes, reverse transcriptase (RT) enzyme [1] and the first human retrovirus, human T-lymphotropic virus type 1 (HTLV-1) [2, 3].

Feline Leukemia Virus (FeLV) was the first retrovirus isolated in domestic cats [4], and the infection is associated with a wide variety of clinical syndromes, including feline acquired immunodeficiency syndrome (AIDS or fAIDS). Since then, the feline AIDS was associated with FeLV, even in animals persistently negative in diagnostic tests [5]. Studies on feline immunosuppressive conditions changed in 1987, after the isolation of another retrovirus in a cat persistently seronegative for FeLV, which progressed to AIDS [6]. This virus was originally called feline T-lymphotropic virus (FTLV). In 1988, it was renamed Feline Immunodeficiency Virus (FIV) [7, 8]. Retrospective studies demonstrated the presence of antibodies anti-FIV in serum samples stored in Japan since 1968 and in the period of 1975-1976 in UK, indicating that the existence of FIV in domestic cats´ population is older than the first description of this virus [9, 10].

EPIDEMIOLOGY

FIV was detected worldwide, with seroprevalence rates between 23% in the US, 10% in southern Europe, 2-6% in northern Europe [11], and 24% in Australia [12]. The highest prevalence rate was recorded in Japan (23.2%) [13]. In Brazil, seroprevalence rates were 14% in São Paulo [14] and 16.66% in Rio de Janeiro [15].

FIV infection is acquired most commonly after 1 year old, and its prevalence increases in animals between 5-10 years. Male cats have a higher risk to become infected than females [16].

These and other variations in the distribution of FIV occurs mainly by differences in social behavior and lifestyle of cats (outdoor versus indoor), which influences the transmission rates of the virus [17].

Classification

FIV is classified in the family Retroviridae, subfamily Orthoretrovirinae, Lentivirus genus, based on its morphology, magnesium-dependent Reverse Transcriptase activity and pathogenesis [18].

Viral Structure

The complete viral particle (virion) has 105-125 nm, spherical shape, and consists of three layers. The outer layer is constituted by an envelope, which is derived from the infected cell membrane during viral budding. The core is involved by a rough spherical matrix, which, in turn, is surrounded by the envelope. The inner layer is composed by an icosahedral capsid involving genome-nucleoprotein complex with helical symmetry. The genomic RNA is highly condensed in the virion by its association with the nucleocapsid protein [18, 19, 20].

Genomic Structure

FIV genome has 9,4kb, and is composed by two linear single stranded RNA molecules with positive polarity. Each monomer has a polyadenylated tail (poly A) at terminal 3' and cap structure at terminal 5' [18].

The integrated proviral DNA consists in *gag*, *pol* and *env* genes flanked by two long terminal repeats – LTRs. The LTRs comprise the 3'-untranslated region (3'-U3), 5'-untranslated region (5'- U5), repeat sequences and regulatory signals that act on integration, transcription and polyadenylation of viral RNA [20, 21].

Gag and *pol* genes encode structural and viral enzymes. The *gag* gene encodes structural proteins such as Matrix (MA), Capsid (CA), and Nucleocapsid (NC). The *pol* gene encodes enzymes Protease (PR), Reverse Transcriptase (RT), Integrase (IN) and dUTPase (DU). The *env* gene encodes glycoproteins of envelope - surface-SU (gp95), and transmembrane-TM (gp38) regions and shows variation in amino acid sequence (Figure 1) [18, 22, 23, 24]. MA protein surrounds the capsid, ensuring the integrity of virion particle. CA p24 protein protects the viral genome. The NC associates with genomic RNA and protects it from digestion by nucleases.

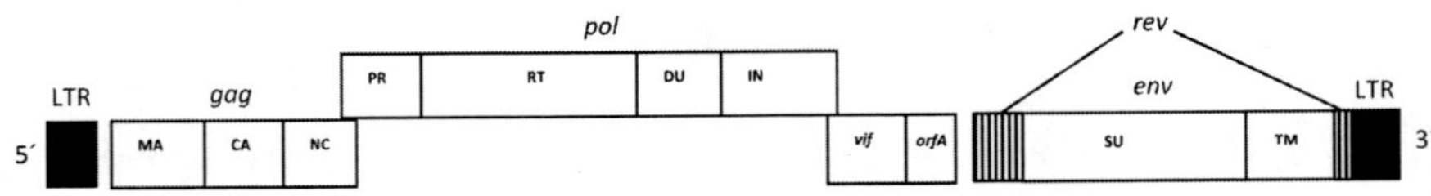

Figure 1. FIV genomic organization. The scheme represents the proviral DNA. Long terminal repeats (LTRs) are located at the extremities of the proviral DNA.Proteins encoded by *gag* gene: MA-matrix, CA-capsid and NC-nucleocapsid. Proteins encoded by *pol* gene: PR-protease, RT-reverse transcriptase, DU-dUTPase, IN-integrase. Proteins encoded by *env* gene: SU-surface and TM-transmembrane. Accessory genes: *vif*, *orfA* and *rev*.

An envelope of host-cell origin surrounds the nucleocapsid. The viral IN catalyzes the incorporation of viral DNA into the host genome [24, 25]. RT is a DNA-dependent RNA polymerase magnesium-dependent, which carries out the reverse transcription of viral RNA into complementary DNA (cDNA) [25]. The PR enzyme is responsible for the processing of polyproteins Gag and Gag-Pol during budding process. This step is essential for infectious viral particle production [26]. The DU catalyzes the conversion of dUTP in dUMP and inorganic pyrophosphate (PPi). The DU activity minimizes the incorporation of dUTP into DNA, which can be mutagenic. DU allows FIV replication in cells in the resting phase, and reduces the frequency of mutations during reverse transcription [18, 27]. Three small open reading frames (ORFs) encode Vif, Orf-A and Rev accessory proteins. Rev protein acts in the transport of unspliced and spliced mRNAs [23]. ORF-A is an apparent transactivator and downregulates CD134, the receptor of FIV [28]. The Vif protein prevents cytidine deamination by cellular deaminase APOBEC 3 [29].

Molecular Characterization

Five subtypes have been identified, A, B, C, D and E [30]. Subtypes A and B are prevalent worldwide (80%), subtype D was identified only in Japan [30, 31, 32] and subtype E was identified in Argentina [33]. Subtype C was described in Vancouver, Munich and Taiwan [34, 35, 36]. Recombinant subtypes A/C, A/B and C/D were found in Canada and Melbourne [37, 38]. The prototype strain Petaluma belongs to subtype A. Subtype B seems to be older and more adapted to the host than other subtypes [34]. In Brazil, subtype B was identified in Minas Gerais, São Paulo and Rio de Janeiro [39, 40, 41], and subtype E was described in Brasilia [42].

Replicative Cycle

The cells initially infected are CD4+ T lymphocytes. With the infection progress, FIV also infects CD8 + T lymphocytes, B lymphocytes, macrophages and cells of the central nervous system [43].

The replication process occurs with the binding of viral Env surface (SU-gp95) and transmembrane (TM-gp38) subunits to the receptor and coreceptor molecules present on the host cell, respectively.

The 43 kDa protein, CD134 (OX40) was described as receptor molecule, and the chemokine receptor CXCR4 as a coreceptor. CD134 is a costimulatory molecule, which expression is restricted to CD4 + lymphocytes in cats, and CXCR4 is widely expressed on activated T cells, B cells and monocytes [43].

After initial interaction, the viral envelope fuses with the cell membrane, releasing the nucleocapsid into the cytoplasm. Still inside the capsid, reverse transcription of single-stranded viral RNA into complementary DNA (cDNA) initiates via viral RT enzyme [44]. The cDNA is transported to the nucleus by viral and cellular proteins, where it integrates into the chromosomal DNA of the host by the action of viral enzyme Integrase.

From this moment, the cDNA is named proviral DNA or provirus and remains throughout life of the infected cell. Therefore, infection persists indefinitely. The provirus may remain dormant or, upon activation, produce viral messenger RNA (mRNA). The viral mRNA migrates into the cytoplasm, and two polyproteins are translated: Gag and Gag-Pol, which are cleaved by viral Protease in the final step of the replicative cycle [26, 44].

The *gag* gene is translated into capsid protein molecules, the *pol* gene into viral enzymes PR, RT, dUTPase and IN, and *env* gene into Env glycoprotein, synthesized as a precursor of 150 kDa. The Env precursor protein goes through the endoplasmic reticulum and is transported to the Golgi complex where it is cleaved into the SU (gp95) and TM (gp38) subunits.

These subunits are conducted to the plasma membrane (PM), where gp38 anchors gp95 to the PM of the infected cell [45]. The polyproteins Gag and Gag-Pol and viral RNA are also addressed to the inner leaflet of the host cell PM, beginning the budding process of nascent virions. The budded virion is immature, since Gag and Gag-Pol precursor polyproteins need to be cleaved by viral PR. The virus matures and becomes ready to infect other cells [46].

Transmission

The main route of transmission is through bites. A high concentration of virus is found in the saliva of infected animals, thereby bites effectively introduce the virus into the bloodstream. Based on the behavior of the species, unsterilized male cats, free-living or living in areas with high population density are considered a risk group [18]. Blood transfusion is another important way of transmission, and blood donors should be tested [47].

Other less common routes in natural infection includes sexual and vertical transmission [48].

Pathogenesis

Natural or experimental disease is characterized by two viremias, which occur at the beginning and end of infection, and a long period of low viral replication. In the initial phase, replication of FIV occurs in CD4+ T lymphocytes, dendritic and macrophages cells. In this phase, about 12 weeks after infection, viral RNA is detected in plasma and proviral DNA in PBMC [49, 50]. Along with viremia, antibodies anti-FIV are detected in plasma, generally 2-4 weeks after infection. Clinical signs are mild, such as anorexia, fever and enlargement of peripheral lymph nodes.

Viral replication is controlled by immune response, plasma viral load is reduced and the infected cat shows no clinical symptoms. This is the asymptomatic stage of the disease, which can last for years. During all stages of the infection a progressive decline in CD4+ T lymphocyte numbers is observed, resulting in a reduced CD4:CD8 T lymphocyte ratio. The progressive immune dysfunction results in FAIDS, the last stage. A new viremic peak is observed; antibody levels decline and infected cats exhibit symptoms of immune deficiency, like opportunistic infections [51, 52].

Infection in newborn feline results in an accelerated progression of the disease, since the developing thymus is a target for viral replication [53].

Immunologic Alterations

Cytokines profile is altered in acute and chronic FIV infection, with decreased interleukin 2 (IL-2), increased IL-6 and tumor necrosis factor alpha

(TNFα) production by peripheral blood mononuclear cells (PBMC), in response to mitogen stimulation [54].

Increased levels of IgG (hypergammaglobulinemia) and impaired neutrophil adhesion and emigration in response to bacterial products were documented in FIV infected cats, as well increased circulating immune complexes, leading to immune complex deposition disorders [54].

CLINICAL AND HEMATOLOGICAL ALTERATIONS

The evolution of disease depends on several factors such as age, immune and health status, dose and route of viral inoculation, and the virus strain.

The clinical signs are generally nonspecific. Clinical and hematological alterations can be related to the direct effects of the virus or to the immunosuppressive effects, which increase the susceptibility to secondary infections and opportunistic agents [55].

FIV is a lentivirus, which means slow virus, because it takes a long time to cause disease. Infection undergoes three phases: acute, asymptomatic and FAIDS. In the acute stage clinical signs are mild and transient, including fever and generalized lymph node enlargement. This stage is followed by an asymptomatic phase, characterized by a long period without symptoms. In kittens, the asymptomatic stage is shortened, especially when they are infected *in utero* or at birth [55, 56]. In the last phase of infection, clinical manifestations of FAIDS occur, such as poor coat condition, diarrhea, fever, weight loss, behavioral and neurological disorders, abscesses, dermatological, respiratory, renal, urinary tract, lung and oral cavity diseases. Opportunistic infections commonly associated include toxoplasmosis, demodicosis, candidiasis, cryptococcosis, mycobacteriosis or Mycoplasma hemofelis/ hemominutum. Neoplasia is directly or indirectly associated with FIV infection, and includes squamous cell carcinoma, fibrosarcoma, mast cell tumor and lymphoma [57, 58, 59, 60]. Chronic stomatitis is the most common syndrome found in natural infection. Lesions are painful, and tooth loss is common. This condition leads to anorexia and emaciation. However, this type of stomatitis is commonly associated with Feline Calicivirus (FCV) [61].

Neurological manifestations were documented in infected cats, and tend to be more behavioral than motor. Even without neurological signs, a higher proportion of infected cats exhibit abnormal forebrain electrical activity, microscopic CNS lesions, and altered visual and auditory evoked potentials [62, 63, 64].

Hematological alterations also vary according to the clinical condition. Anemia, lymphocytosis or lymphopenia, neutropenia and thrombocytopenia are commonly associated with FIV infection. Cytopenias, mainly neutropenia and lymphopenia, in general are correlated with immunosupression [65].

Cats in the asymptomatic stage usually do not show hematologic abnormalities [65].

DIAGNOSIS

Serological Tests

Cats infected by FIV develop high levels of antibodies against FIV proteins about four weeks post infection, and the presence of antibodies is correlated with persistent infection [66, 67].

Several methods are available to detect these antibodies, although veterinary practitioners commonly use serological in house assays. Rapid immunochromatography and ELISA tests are highly sensitivity and specific, easily performed and faster, lasting usually 10 minutes to read the results.

These tests are combined to detect simultaneously antibodies against FIV proteins (usually p24 capsid protein and/or gp38 transmembrane protein) and FeLV p27 (capsid protein) antigen. ELISA test in reference laboratory is performed using a micro titer plate format.

Western blot (WB) test detect antibodies against at least two structural FIV proteins, p15 and p24, being more specific than ELISA or immunochromatography tests, and is selected for confirmation of infection following positive ELISA result [47].

Polymerase Chain Reaction (PCR)

PCR is a very sensitive and specific method that can be used to detect FIV proviral DNA in peripheral blood mononuclear cells (PBMC) or viral RNA in plasma. The detection of proviral DNA indicates that the virus has entered the cell and its genome is integrated into the cell host.

Detection of viral RNA indicates viral production. Real-time PCR (qPCR) is a more sensitive and specific variation of this method that allows detection and quantitation of proviral or viral load [52, 68, 69, 70, 71].

PCR is a useful method for early detection, since FIV provirus is detected 6 to 8 weeks post infection in experimental infection studies, while serological methods takes about four months to identify an infected cat [71, 72, 73, 74].

Viral Culture

Virus cultivation is a reliable way to detect infectious virus, but is laborious and the result is obtained in two to three weeks. Therefore, this test is not considered for routine [47].

Discordant Results

Discordant results using serological methods (ELISA, immunochromatography, WB) are possible due to the evolution of infection, cross-reactions or in some specific situations.

Serological tests can detect maternal antibodies in kittens less than 6 months of age, generating a false positive result. Kittens should be tested again after 6 months of age, and considered true positive if antibody tests remain positive. The queen should be tested in parallel to ensure the immunological status [47].

False negative results are possible in animals that do not realize seroconversion, when serological test is performed before seroconversion (soon after exposure - i.e. bites) or in terminal stages of disease, since the cat is immunosuppressed [47, 74].

Cross-reactions leading to false positive serological tests may occur in tests using viral antigens gradient-purified, because they contain components of the cell in which the virus is propagated. Viral vaccines developed in cell culture also induce this type of response. Therefore, cats routinely vaccinated against other viral diseases may cross-react in serological tests [18, 75].

Antibody based tests cannot discriminate antibodies from cats vaccinated with a FIV vaccine versus antibodies from true infection. PCR is a useful method to distinguish in this case [76].

Discordant results with PCR methods may be obtained due to variations in FIV strain or to the sensitivity of method, when provirus DNA or viral RNA are below the threshold needed for detection (false negative results) [76, 77]. False positive results might occur by contamination of reaction or unspecific primer binding.

Inconclusive tests may be elucidated using an alternate method [50, 78].

All tests can be accomplished using whole blood; however, serum samples are preferred for FIV antibodies screening. PCR tests can also be done using saliva, since a high number of viral particles are detected in this fluid [77].

Kittens and adult cats should be tested when adopted. Cats at higher risk for infection, for example cats with outdoor habits or living with cats which might be infected, should be yearly tested [47].

TREATMENT

Since there is no cure for infected cats, the goal of treatment is to control clinical conditions. For the treatment of symptomatic and opportunistic infections, bactericidal antibiotics are necessary, as the immune system of the infected cat is compromised. In this context, the use of immunomodulators has been widely used, with satisfactory results [47].

Interferons (IFNs) are cytokines expressed in response to stimulation of a variety of receptors that recognize pathogens, and they were described as antiviral factors. Human or feline IFN is used to treat FIV infected cats [78].

It was demonstrated that low oral doses of human alpha IFN enhances immune response for viral infections, with modulation of cytokines IL-1, IL-5, IL-6, IL-8. This approach has been utilized to treat infected cats. The low oral dose (10IU/kg) of natural human alpha interferon showed more significant clinical improvement than the treatment with recombinant human alpha IFN. However, low dose (30IU/cat) of recombinant human alpha IFN is normally used in a daily regimen for 7 days on, 7 days off [47, 78, 79].

The chronic use of human interferon in cats can induce antibodies development with loss of its efficacy. However, since alpha IFN is degraded by proteolytic enzymes after oral treatment, it is not detected in the systemic circulation [78].

Recombinant feline omega interferon (Virbagen®, Virbac- a type-I IFN) was licensed to veterinary use in Europe, Japan, Australia, New Zealand and Mexico, and treated cats presented clinical improved and increased survival rates. The treatment schedule consists of subcutaneous administration of 1 MU/kg/day for five consecutive days in three separated treatments at day 0, day 14 and day 60. Oral treatment with 0.1 MU/cat once a day is also possible [80, 81]. Antiretroviral therapy (ARV) was developed to control HIV-1 replication. Different steps of HIV replicative cycle have been targeted for the development of compounds with antiretroviral activity [82].

These compounds were divided in four classes: RT inhibitors, protease inhibitors, integrase inhibitors and fusion/entry inhibitors [83]. Due to similarities between HIV and FIV, some of these classes of drugs have been tested to control FIV. Several of them proved to be toxic to cats and do not inhibit FIV, e.g. protease inhibitors (PI) [84].

The nucleoside RT inhibitors (NRTIs) Zidovudine (AZT) and Lamivudine (3TC) were the first anti-HIV drugs approved by the Food and Drug Administration (FDA) and they work synergistically [85]. These drugs were the most studied to control FIV *in vitro* and *in vivo*, alone or in combination. Data about doses and clinical use vary and are contradictory [86, 87, 88]. Despite this, AZT is the only antiretroviral recommended by the European Advisory Committee for Diseases of Cats (European Advisory Board on Cat Diseases - ABCD) at a dose of 5 mg/kg every 12 hours. Monitoring of hematological parameters is indicated due to the main side effect of AZT, such as anemia development. Treatment should be discontinued if the hematocrit falls below 20%. Hematocrit values return to normal after discontinuation of the drug [47]. Despite the anemia due to AZT, there is an adaptation of the bone marrow with the continued use [88]. 3TC monotherapy (25mg/kg/PO/q 12h) is used instead of AZT, since it is considered a safer drug, with little side effects [89].

Renal clearance is the major route of AZT and 3TC elimination, so a dose reduction or discontinuation of the drug is indicated in cats with renal disease [90, 91].

Other components are under study, with promising results. Recent *in vitro* studies showed a good response to FIV integrase inhibitors and with protease inhibitor tipranavir [92, 93]. *In vivo* tests were done with acyclic nucleoside phosphonates (S)-9-(3-fluoro-2-phosphonylmethoxypropyl) adenine (FPMPA) and 9-(2-phosphonylmethoxyethyl) adenine (PMEA) and demonstrated effectiveness in the improvement of clinical symptoms of FIV-infected cats.

The nucleoside analogue (R)-9-(2-phosphonylmethoxypropyl)-2,6-diaminopurine (PMPDAP), a congener of FPMPA, was used to treat cats naturally infected in a regimen of 25 mg/kg subcutaneously twice a week, with good results [94, 95]. Despite this, further investigations are necessary.

AMD3100 (Plerixafor) is another promising drug that acts as a FIV entry inhibitor. This drug, not approved as antiviral, acts as a selective antagonist of FIV coreceptor, CXCR4 and inhibits virus entry. A study in naturally infected cats showed that treatment with AMD3100 (0.5 mg/kg q12h SC for 6 weeks) reduced the clinical signs and proviral load with no reported side effects [96].

Viral resistance to ARVs is a limiting factor with long-term monotherapy [97]. According to reports of veterinary practitioners, the viral resistance to ARVs seems to occur late in cats with FIV. Symptomatic cats showed clinical improvement for periods longer than one year whith the use of AZT or 3TC monotherapy.

PREVENTION

The main prevention measures include spaying and keep the cat indoors; new cats should be tested before being introduced into a multi-cat household and re-tested after quarantine period of at least 6 weeks [47, 73].

A FIV vaccine is available in the US, Australia and New Zealand. This is an inactivated vaccine with efficiency of 82%, composed by subtypes A and D isolate from long-term nonprogressors (LTNP) cats. However, serological tests do not differentiate vaccinated from infected cats [98, 99, 100].

REFERENCES

[1] Coffin, J. M., Hughes, S. H., Varmus, H. E. The Interactions of Retroviruses and their Hosts. In: Coffin, J. M., Hughes, S. H., Varmus, H. E., editors. *Retroviruses*. Cold Spring Harbor (NY): Cold Spring Harbor Laboratory Press; 1997.

[2] Poiesz, B. J., Ruscetti, F. W., Gazdar, A. F., Bunn, P. A., Minna, J. D., Gallo, R. C. (1980). Detection and isolation of type C retrovirus particles from fresh and cultured lymphocytes of a patient with cutaneous T-cell lymphoma. *Proceedings of the National Academy of Sciences of the United States of America*. 77 (12): 7415-7419.

[3] Gallo, R. C. (2005). The discovery of the first human retrovirus: HTLV-1 and HTLV-2. *Retrovirology*. 2 (1): 1-7.

[4] Jarrett, W. F., Crawford, E. M., Martin, W. B., Davie, F. (1964). A virus-like particle associated with leukemia (lymphosarcoma). *Nature* 9 (202):567-569.

[5] Hagiwara, M. K. (1990). AIDS felina. *Ciência Hoje*; 12 (68): 62-64.

[6] Pedersen, N. C., Ho, E. W., Brown, M. L. (1987). Isolation of a T-lymphotropic virus from domestic cats with a immunodeficiency-like syndrome. *Science*. 235 (4790): 790-793.

[7] Sparger, E. E. (1993). Current thoughts on feline immunodeficiency virus infection. The Veterinary Clinics of North America. *Small Animal Practice.* 23 (1): 173-191.

[8] Yamamoto, J. K., Pedersen, N. C., Ho, E. W., Okuda, T., Theilen, G. H. (1988). Feline immunodeficiency syndrome--a comparison between feline T-lymphotropic lentivirus and feline leukemia virus. *Leukemia.* 2 (12 Suppl.): 204S-215S.

[9] Furuya, T., Kawaguchi, Y., Miyazawa, T., Fujikawa, Y., Tohya, Y., Azetaka, M., Takahashi, E., Mikami, T. (1990). Existence of feline immunodeficiency virus infection in Japanese cat population since 1968. *Japanese Journal of Veterinary Science* 52 (4): 891-893.

[10] Gruffydd-Jones, T. J., Hopper, C. D., Harbour, D. A., Lutz, H. (1988). Serological evidence of feline immunodeficiency virus infection in UK cats from 1975-76. *Veterinary Record* 123 (22): 569-570.

[11] Gleich, S. E., Krieger, S., Hartmann, K. (2009). Prevalence of feline immunodeficiency virus and feline leukemia virus among client-owned cats and risk factors for infection in Germany. *Journal of Feline Medicine and Surgery* 11:985-992.

[12] Norris, J. M., Bell, E. T., Hales, L., Toribio, J. A., White, J. D., Wigney, D. I., Baral, R. M., Malik, R. (2007). Prevalence of feline immunodeficiency virus infection in domesticated and feral cats in eastern Australia. *Journal of Feline Medicine and Surgery* 9 (4):300-308.

[13] Nakamura, Y., Nakamura, Y., Ura, A., Hirata, M., Sakuma, M., Sakata, Y., Nishigaki, K., Tsujimoto, H., Setoguchi, A., Endo, Y. (2010). An updated nation-wide epidemiological survey of feline immunodeficiency virus (FIV) infection in Japan. *Journal of Veterinary Medical Science* 72 (8):1051-1056.

[14] Reche Jr. A., Hagiwara, M. K., Lucas, S. R. R. (1997). Clinical study of acquired immunodeficiency syndrome in domestic cats in São Paulo. *Brazilian Journal of Veterinary Research and Animal Science* 34(3): 152-155.

[15] Souza, H. J. M., Graça, R. F. S., Teixeira, C. H. R. (2002). Estudo epidemiológico das infecções pelos vírus da leucemia e/ou imunodeficiência felina em gatos domésticos do município do Rio de Janeiro. *Clínica Veterinária*. 36:14-21.

[16] Levy, J. K., Scott, H. M., Lachtara, J. L., Crawford, P. C. (2006). Seroprevalence of feline leucemia virus and feline immunodeficiency virus infection among cats in North America and risk factors for

seropositivity. *Journal of American Veterinary Medical Association* 228 (3):371-376.

[17] Bahi-Jaber, N., Langlais, M., Pontier, D. (2003). Behavioral plasticity and virus propagation: the FIV-cat population example. *Theoretical Population Biology* 64(1): 11-24.

[18] Bendinelli, M., Pistello, M., Lombardi, S., Poli, A., Garzelli, C., Matteucci, D., et al. (1995). Feline Immunodeficiency Virus: an interesting model for AIDS studies and an important cat pathogen. *Clinical Microbiology Reviews*. 8 (1): 87-112.

[19] Pedersen, N. C., Yamamoto, J. K., Ishida, T., Hansen, H. (1989). Feline immunodeficiency virus infection. *Veterinary Immunology and Immunopathology* 21(1):111-129.

[20] Tomonaga, K. and Mikami, T. (1996). Molecular biology of the feline immunodeficiency virus auxiliary genes. *Journal of General Virology* 77 (Pt 8):1611-1621.

[21] Elder, J. H., Sundstrom, M., de Rozieres, S., de Parseval, A., Grant, C. K., Lin, Y. C. (2008). Molecular mechanisms of FIV infection. *Veterinary Immunology and Immunopathology* 123(1-2):3-13.

[22] Miyazawa, T. and Mikami, T. (1993). Biological nature of feline immunodeficiency virus. *Journal of Veterinary Medical Science* 55(4): 519-526.

[23] Miyazawa, T., Tomonaga, K., Kawaguchi, Y., Mikami, T. (1994). The genome of feline immunodeficiency virus. *Archives of Virology* 134: 221-234.

[24] Caxito, F. A., Resende, M. (2004). Feline immunodeficiency virus: a review. *Virus Reviews and Research*. 2 (9): 7-17.

[25] O'Reilly, M. M., McNally, M. T., Beemon, K. L. (1995). Two strong 5' splice sites and competing, suboptimal 3' splice sites involved in alternative splicing of human immunodeficiency virus type 1 RNA. *Virology* 213(2):373-385.

[26] Lin, Y. C., Beck, Z., Morris, G. M., Olson, A. J., Elder, J. H. (2003). Structural basis for distinctions between substrate and inhibitor specificities for feline immunodeficiency virus and human immunodeficiency virus proteases. *Journal of Virology*. 77 (12): 6589-6600.

[27] Miller, R. J., Cairns, J. S., Bridges, S., Sarver, N. (2000). Minireview – Human Immunodeficiency Virus and AIDS: Insights from Animal Lentiviruses. *Journal of Virology*. 74 (16): 7187-7195.

[28] Hong, Y., Fink, E., Hu, Q. Y., Kiosses, W. B., Elder, J. H. (2010). OrfA downregulates feline immunodeficiency virus primary receptor CD134 on the host cell surface and is important in viral infection. *Journal of Virology* 84(14):7225-7232.

[29] Troyer, R. M., Thompson, J., Elder, J. H., VandeWoude, S. (2013). Accessory genes confer a high replication rate to virulent feline immunodeficiency virus. *Journal of Virology* 87(14):7940-7951.

[30] Sodora, D. L., Shpaer, E. G., Kitchell, B. E., Dow, S. W., Hoover, E. A., Mullins, J. I. (1994). Identification of three feline immunodeficiency virus (FIV) env gene subtypes and comparison of the FIV and human immunodeficiency virus type 1 evolutionary patterns. *Journal of Virology*. 68 (4): 2230-2238.

[31] Samman, A., McMonagle, E. L., Logan, N., Willett, B. J., Biek, R., Hosie, M. J. (2011). Phylogenetic characterisation of naturally occurring feline immunodeficiency virus in the United Kingdom. *Veterinary Microbiology* 150(3-4):239-247.

[32] Kakinuma, S., Motokawa, K., Hohdatsu, T., Yamamoto, J. K., Koyama, H., Hashimoto, H. (1995). Nucleotide sequence of feline immunodeficiency virus: classification of japanese isolates into two subtypes which are distinct from non-japanese subtypes. *Journal of Virology* 69 (6): 3639-3646.

[33] Pecoraro, M. R., Tomonaga, K., Miyazawa, T., Kawaguchi, Y., Sugita, S., Tohya, Y., Kai, C., Etcheverrigaray, M. E., Mikami, T. (1996). Genetic diversity of Argentine isolates of feline immunodeficiency virus. *Journal of General Virology*. 77 (Pt 9): 2031-2035.

[34] Sodora, D. L., Shpaer, E. G., Kitchell, B. E., Dow, S. W., Hoover, E. A., Mullins, J. I. (1994). Identification of three feline immunodeficiency virus (FIV) env gene subtypes and comparison of the FIV and human immunodeficiency virus type 1 evolutionary patterns. *Journal of Virology*. 68 (4): 2230-2238.

[35] Bachmann, M. H., Mathiason-Dubard, C., Learn, G. H., Rodrigo, A. G., Sodora, D. L., Mazzetti, P., Hoover, E. A., Mullins, J. I. (1997). Genetic diversity of feline immunodeficiency virus: dual infection, recombination, and distinct evolutionary rates among envelope sequence clades. *Journal of Virology*; 71 (6): 4241-4253.

[36] Inada, G., Miyazawa, T., Inoshima, Y., Kohmoto, M., Ikeda, Y., Liu, C. H., Lin, J. A., Kuo, T. F., Mikami, T. (1997). Phylogenetic analysis of feline immunodeficiency virus isolated from cats in Taiwan. *Archives of Virology*. 142 (7): 1459-1467.

[37] Reggeti, F., Bienzle, D. (2004). Feline immunodeficiency virus subtypes A, B and C and intersubtype recombinants in Ontario, Canada. *Journal of General Virology* 85:1843-1852.

[38] Iwata, D., Holloway, S. A. (2008). Molecular subtyping of feline immunodeficiency virus from cats in Melbourne. *Australian Veterinary Journal* 86(10):385-389.

[39] Caxito, F. A., Coelho, F. M., Oliveira, M. E., Resende, M. (2006). Feline immunodeficiency virus subtype B in domestic cats in Minas Gerais, Brazil. *Veterinary Research Communications* 30(8):953-956.

[40] Lara, V. M., Taniwaki, S. A., Araújo, Jr J. P. (2007). Caracterização filogenética de amostras do Vírus da Imunodeficiência Felina (FIV) do Estado de São Paulo. *Pesquisa Veterinária Brasileira* 27: 467-470.

[41] Martins, A. N., Medeiros, S. O., Simonetti, J. P., Schatzmayr, H. G., Tanuri, A., Brindeiro, R. M. (2008). Phylogenetic and genetic analysis of feline immunodeficiency virus *gag*, *pol*, and *env* genes from domestic cats undergoing nucleoside reverse transcriptase inhibitor treatment or treatment-naïve cats in Rio de Janeiro, Brazil. *Journal of Virology* 82 (16):7863-7874.

[42] Marçola, T. G., Gomes, C. P., Silva, P. A., Fernandes, G. R., Paludo, G. R., Pereira, R. W. (2013). Identification of a novel subtype of feline immunodeficiency virus in a population of naturally infected felines in the Brazilian Federal District. *Virus Genes* 46(3):546-550.

[43] Shimojima, M., Miyazawa, T., Ikeda, Y., McMonagle, E. L., Haining, H., Akashi, H., Takeuchi, Y., Hosie, M. J., Willett, B. J. (2004). Use of CD134 as a primary receptor by the feline immunodeficiency virus. *Science*. 303 (5661): 1192-1195.

[44] Kanzaki, L. I., Looney, D. J. (2004). Feline immunodeficiency virus: a concise review. *Frontiers in Bioscience* 9: 370-377.

[45] Verschoor, E. J., Hulskotte, E. G., Ederveen, J., Koolen, M. J., Horzinek, M. C., Rottier, P. J. (1993). Post-translational processing of the feline immunodeficiency virus envelope precursor protein. *Virology*. 193 (1): 433-438.

[46] Elder, J. H., Schnolzer, M., Hasselkus-Light, C. S., Henson, M., Lerner, D. A., Phillips, T. R., Wagaman, P. C., Kent, S. B. (1993). Identification of proteolytic processing sites within the gag and pol polyproteins of feline immunodeficiency virus. *Journal of Virology*, 67(4), 1869–1876.

[47] Hosie, M. J., Addie, D., Belák, S., et al. (2009). Feline immunodeficiency. ABCD guidelines on prevention and management. *Journal of feline medicine and surgery* 11:575–584.

[48] Medeiros, S. O., Martins, A. N., Dias, C. G., Tanuri, A., Brindeiro, R. M. (2012). Natural transmission of feline immunodeficiency virus from infected queen to kitten. *Virology Journal* 9:99.
[49] Beebe, A. M., Dua, N., Faith, T. G., Moore, P. F., Pedersen, N. C., Dandekar, S. (1994). Primary stage of feline immunodeficiency virus infection: viral dissemination and cellular targets. *Journal of Virology* 68 (5):3080-3091.
[50] Obert, L. A. and Hoover, E. A. (2002). Early pathogenesis of transmucosal feline immunodeficiency virus infection. *Journal of Virology* 76(12):6311-6322.
[51] Diehl, L. J., Mathiason-Dubard, C. K., O'Neil, L. L., Hoover, E. A. (1996). Plasma viral RNA load predicts disease progression in accelerated feline immunodeficiency virus infection. *Journal of Virology* 70(4):2503-2507.
[52] Goto, Y., Nishimura, Y., Baba, K., Mizuno, T., Endo, Y., Masuda, K., Ohno, K., Tsujimoto, H. (2002). Association of plasma viral RNA load with prognosis in cats naturally infected with feline immunodeficiency virus. *Journal of Virology* 76(19):10079-10083.
[53] Kolenda-Roberts, H. M., Kuhnt, L. A., Jennings, R. N., Mergia, A., Gengozian, N., Johnson, C. M. (2007). Immunopathogenesis of feline immunodeficiency virus infection in the fetal and neonatal cat. *Frontiers in Bioscience* 1 (12)3668-3682.
[54] Burkhard, M. J. and Dean, G. A. (2003). Transmission and immunopathogenesis of FIV in cats as a model for HIV. *Current HIV Research* 1(1):15-29.
[55] Callanan, J. J., Thompson, H., Toth, S. R., O'Neil, B., Lawrence, C. E., Willett, B., Jarrett, O. (1992). Clinical and pathological findings in feline immunodeficiency virus experimental infection. *Veterinary Immunology and Immunopathology.* 35 (1-2):3-13.
[56] Rogers, A. B. and Hoover, E. A. (2002). Fetal feline immunodeficiency virus is prevalent and occult. *Journal of Infectious Diseases* 186:895-904.
[57] Beatty, J. A., Lawrence, C. E., Callanan, J. J., Grant, C. K., Gault, E. A., Neil, J. C., Jarrett, O. (1998). Feline immunodeficiency virus (FIV)-associated lymphoma: a potential role for immune dysfunction in tumourigenesis. *Veterinary Immunology and Immunopathology* 65(2-4): 309-322.
[58] Wang, J., Kyaw-Tanner, M., Lee, C., Robinson, W. F. (2001). Characterisation of lymphosarcomas in Australian cats using polymerase

chain reaction and immunohistochemical examination. *Australian Veterinary Journal* 79(1):41-46.

[59] Terry, A., Callanan, J. J., Fulton, R., Jarrett, O., Neil, J. C. (1995). Molecular analysis of tumours from feline immunodeficiency virus (FIV)-infected cats: an indirect role for FIV? *International Journal of Cancer* 61(2):227-232.

[60] Gabor, L. J., Love, D. N., Malik, R., Canfield, P. J. (2001). Feline immunodeficiency virus status of Australian cats with lymphosarcoma. *Australian Veterinary Journal* 79(8):540-545.

[61] Tenorio, A. P., Franti, C. E., Madewell, B. R., Pedersen, N. C. (1991). Chronic oral infections of cats and their relationship to persistent oral carriage of feline calici-, immunodeficiency, or leukemia viruses. *Veterinary Immunology Immunopathology* 29(1-2):1-14.

[62] Podell, M., Oglesbee, M., Mathes, L., Krakowka, S., Olmstead, R., Lafrado, L. (1993). AIDS-associated encephalopathy with experimental feline immunodeficiency virus infection. *Journal of Acquired Immune Deficiency Syndrome* 6(7):758-771.

[63] Gómez, N. V., Fontanals, A., Castillo, V., Gisbert, M. A., Suraniti, A., Mira, G., Pisano, P. B. (2012). Evaluation of different antiretroviral drug protocols on naturally infected feline immunodeficiency virus (FIV) cats in the late phase of the asymptomatic stage of infection. *Viruses* 4(6): 924-939.

[64] Pistello, M., Moscardini, M., Mazzetti, P., Bonci, F., Zaccaro, L., Isola, P., Freer, G., Specter, S., Matteucci, D., Bendinelli, M. (2002). Development of feline immunodeficiency virus ORF-A (tat) mutants: in vitro and in vivo characterization. *Virology* 298(1):84-95.

[65] Gleich, S., Hartmann, K. (2009). Hematology and serum biochemistry of feline immunodeficiency virus-infected and feline leukemia virus-infected cats. *Journal of Veterinary Internal Medicine* 23(3):552-558.

[66] Egberink, H. F., Keldermans, C. E. J. M., Koolen, M. J. M., Horzinek, M. C. (1992). Humoral immune response to feline immunodeficiency virus in cats with experimentally induced and naturally acquired infections. *American Journal of Veterinary Research* 53 (7):1133-1138.

[67] Wood, B. A., Carver, S., Troyer, R. M., Elder, J. H., VandeWoude, S. (2013). Domestic cat microsphere immunoassays: detection of antibodies during feline immunodeficiency virus infection. *Journal of Immunological Methods* 396(1-2):74-86.

[68] Lawson, M., Meers, J., Blechynden, L., Robinson, W., Greene, W., Carnegie, P. (1993). The detection and quantification of feline

immunodeficiency provirus in peripheral blood mononuclear cells using the polymerase chain reaction. *Veterinary Microbiology* 38(1-2):11-21.

[69] Hohdatsu, T., Yamada, M., Okada, M., Fukasawa, M., Watanabe, K., Ogasawara, T., Takagi, M., Aizawa, C., Hayami, M., Koyama, H. (1992). Detection of feline immunodeficiency proviral DNA in peripheral blood lymphocytes by the polymerase chain reaction. *Veterinary Microbiology* 30(2-3):113-123.

[70] Heid, C. A., Stevens, J., Livak, K. J., Williams, P. M. (1996). Real time quantitative PCR. *Genome Research* 6(10):986-994.

[71] Pedersen, N. C., Leutenegger, C. M., Woo, J., Higgins, J. (2001). Virulence differences between two field isolates of feline immunodeficiency virus (FIV-A Petaluma and FIV-CPGammar) in young adult specific pathogen free cats. *Veterinary Immunology and Immunopathology* 79(1-2):53-67.

[72] Dua, N., Reubel, G., Moore, P. F., Higgins, J., Pedersen, N. C. (1994). An experimental study of primary feline immunodeficiency virus infection in cats and a historical comparison to acute simian and human immunodeficiency virus diseases. *Veterinary Immunology and Immunopathology* 43(4):337-355.

[73] Möstl, K., Egberink, H., Addie, D., Frymus, T., Boucraut-Baralon, C., Truyen, U., Hartmann, K., Lutz, H., Gruffydd-Jones, T., Radford, A. D., Lloret, A., Pennisi, M. G., Hosie, M. J., Marsilio, F., Thiry, E., Belák, S., Horzinek, M. C. (2013). Prevention of infectious diseases in cat shelters: ABCD guidelines. *Journal of Feline Medicine and Surgery* 15(7):546-554.

[74] Dandekar, S., Beebe, A. M., Barlough, J., Phillips, T., Elder, J., Torten, M., Pedersen, N. (1992). Detection of feline immunodeficiency virus (FIV) nucleic acids in FIV-seronegative cats. *Journal of Virology* 66(7): 4040-4049.

[75] Calandrella, M., Matteucci, D., Mazzetti, P., Poli, A. (2001). Densitometric analysis of Western blot assays for feline immunodeficiency virus antibodies. *Veterinary Immunology and Immunopathology* 79(3-4):261-271.

[76] Ammersbach, M., Little, S., Bienzle, D. (2013). Preliminary evaluation of a quantitative polymerase chain reaction assay for diagnosis of feline immunodeficiency virus infection. *Journal of Feline Medicine and Surgery.* 15(8):725-729.

[77] Matteucci, D., Baldinotti, F., Mazzetti, P., Pistello, M., Bandecchi, P., Ghilarducci, R., Poli, A., Tozzini, F., Bendinelli, M. (1993). Detection of

feline immunodeficiency virus in saliva and plasma by cultivation and polymerase chain reaction. *Journal of Clinical Microbiology* 31(3):494-501.

[78] Gómez, N. V., Castillo, V. A., Gisbert, M. A., Pisano, P., Mira, G., Fontanals, A., Blatter, M. F. (2011). Immune-endocrine interactions in treated and untreated cats naturally infected with FIV. *Veterinary Immunology and Immunopathology* 143(3-4):332-337.

[79] Pedretti, E., Passeri, B., Amadori, M., Isola, P., Di Pede, P., Telera, A., Vescovini, R., Quintavalla, F., Pistello, M. (2006). Low-dose interferon-alpha treatment for feline immunodeficiency virus infection. *Veterinary Immunology and Immunopathology* 109(3-4):245-254.

[80] Gil, S., Leal, R. O., Duarte, A., McGahie, D., Sepúlveda, N., Siborro, I., Cravo, J., Cartaxeiro, C., Tavares, L. M. (2013). Relevance of feline interferon omega for clinical improvement and reduction of concurrent viral excretion in retrovirus infected cats from a rescue shelter. *Research in Veterinary Science* 94(3):753-763.

[81] Gil, S., Leal, R. O., McGahie, D., Sepúlveda, N., Duarte, A., Niza, M. M., Tavares, L. (2014). Oral Recombinant Feline Interferon-Omega as an alternative immune modulation therapy in FIV positive cats: clinical and laboratory evaluation. *Research in Veterinary Science* 96(1):79-85.

[82] Brigido, L., Rodrigues, R., Casseb, J., Custodio, R. M., Fonseca, L. A., Sanchez, M., Duarte, A. J. (2004). CD4+ T-cell recovery and clinical outcome in HIV-1-infected patients exposed to multiple antiretroviral regimens: partial control of viremia is associated with favorable outcome. *AIDS Patient Care and STDs*. 18(4):189-198.

[83] De Clercq, E. (2009). Anti-HIV drugs: 25 compounds approved within 25 years after the discovery of HIV. *International Journal of Antimicrobial Agents.* 33(4):307-320.

[84] Auwerx, J., Esnouf, R., De Clercq, E., Balzarini, J. (2004). Susceptibility of feline immunodeficiency virus/human immunodeficiency virus type 1 reverse transcriptase chimeras to non-nucleoside RT inhibitors. *Molecular Pharmacology* 65:244–251.

[85] Eron, J. J. (1995). Treatment with Lamivudine, Zidovudine, or Both in HIV-Positive Patients with 200 to 500 CD4+ Cells per Cubic Millimeter. *New England Journal of Medicine* 333:1662–1669.

[86] Hartmann, K., Donath, A., Beer, B., et al. (1992). Use of two virustatica (AZT, PMEA) in the treatment of FIV and of FeLV seropositive cats with clinical symptoms. *Veterinary Immunology and Immunopathology* 35:167-175.

[87] Arai, M., Earl, D. D., Yamamoto, J. K. (2002). Is AZT/3TC therapy effective against FIV infection or immunopathogenesis? *Veterinary Immunology and Immunopathology* 85: 189-204.
[88] Hart, S., Nolte, I. (1995). Long-term treatment of disease, FIV-seropositive field cats with azidothymidine (AZT). Zentralblatt für Veterinärmedizin. *Reihe A* 42(6):397-409.
[89] Zhang, W., Mauldin, J. K., Schmiedt, C. W., Brockus, C. W., Boudinot, F. D., McCrackin, S. M. (2004). Pharmacokinetics of lamivudine in cats. *American Journal of Veterinary Research* 65(6):841-846.
[90] Rachlis, A. R. (1990). Zidovudine (Retrovir) update. *Canadian Medical Association Journal* 143(11):1177-1185.
[91] Johnson, M. A., Verpooten, G. A., Daniel, M. J., Plumb, R., Moss, J., Van Caesbroeck, D., De Broe, M. E. (1998). Single dose pharmacokinetics of lamivudine in subjects with impaired renal function and the effect of haemodialysis. *British Journal of Clinical Pharmacology* 46(1):21-27.
[92] Savarino, A., Pistello, M., D'Ostilio, D., Zabogli, E., Taglia, F., Mancini, F., Ferro, S., Matteucci, D., De Luca, L., Barreca, M. L., Ciervo, A., Chimirri, A., Ciccozzi, M., Bendinelli, M. (2007). Human immunodeficiency virus integrase inhibitors efficiently suppress feline immunodeficiency virus replication in vitro and provide a rationale to redesign antiretroviral treatment for feline AIDS. *Retrovirology* 4:79.
[93] Norelli, S., El Daker, S., D'Ostilio, D., Mele, F., Mancini, F., Taglia, F., Ruggieri, A., Ciccozzi, M., Cauda, R., Ciervo, A., Barreca, M. L., Pistello, M., Bendinelli, M., Savarino, A. (2008). Response of feline immunodeficiency virus (FIV) to tipranavir may provide new clues for development of broad-based inhibitors of retroviral proteases acting on drug-resistant HIV-1. *Current HIV Research* 6(4):306-317.
[94] Vahlenkamp, T. W., De Ronde, A., Balzarini, J., Naesens, L., De Clercq, E., van Eijk, M. J., Horzinek, M. C., Egberink, H. F. (1995). (R)-9-(2-phosphonylmethoxypropyl)-2,6-diaminopurine is a potent inhibitor of feline immunodeficiency virus infection. *Antimicrobial Agents and Chemotherapy* 39(3):746-749.
[95] Hartmann, A. D., Wilhelm, N., Balzarini, J., Hartmann, K. (2012). Clinical efficacy of the acyclic nucleoside phosphonate 9-(2-phosphonylmethoxypropyl)-2,6-diaminopurine (PMPDAP) in the treatment of feline immunodeficiency virus-infected cats. *Journal of Feline Medicine and Surgery* 14(2):107-112.

[96] Hartmann, K., Stengel, C., Klein, D., Egberink, H., Balzarini, J. (2012). Efficacy and adverse effects of the antiviral compound plerixafor in feline immunodeficiency virus-infected cats. *Journal of Veterinary Internal Medicine* 26(3):483-490.

[97] Larder, B. A., Kemp, S. D., Purifoy, D. J. (1989). Infectious potential of human immunodeficiency virus type 1 reverse transcriptase mutants with altered inhibitor sensitivity. *Proceedings of the National Academy of Sciences of the United States of America* 86(13):4803-4807.

[98] Pu, R., Coleman, J., Omori, M., Arai, M., Hohdatsu, T., Huang, C., Tanabe, T., Yamamoto, J. K. (2001). Dual-subtype FIV vaccine protects cats against in vivo swarms of both homologous and heterologous subtype FIV isolates. *AIDS* 15 (10): 1225-1237.

[99] Uhl, E. W., Heaton-Jones, T. G., Pu, R., Yamamoto, J. K. (2002). FIV vaccine development and its importance to veterinary and human medicine: a review FIV vaccine 2002 update and review. *Veterinary Immunology and Immunopathology.* 90 (3-4):113-132.

[100] Litster, A., Lin, J. M., Nichols, J., Weng, H. Y. (2014). Diagnostic utility of CD4%:CD8 low% T-lymphocyte ratio to differentiate feline immunodeficiency virus (FIV)-infected from FIV-vaccinated cats. *Veterinary Microbiology* 170(3-4):197-205.

In: Felines
Editor: Colleen Kevins
ISBN: 978-1-63463-550-9

Chapter 4

FELINE ORAL DISEASES

Rita de Cassia da Silva Costa
Universidade Federal Rural do Rio de Janeiro

ABSTRACT

Inflammatory diseases of the oral cavity are common feline medical conditions and are associated with infectious agents such as Feline Immunodeficiency Virus (FIV), Feline Leukemia Virus (FeLV), herpesvirus (FHV-1) and calicivirus (FCV). The most common oral diseases in cats are gingivostomatitis, periodontal disease, tooth resorption and chronic periapical lesion by the canine tooth fracture. Feline gingivostomatitis is characterized by severe and chronic inflammation of gingiva and oral mucosa. The viral and immunological involvement in the pathogenesis of this disease has been increasingly recognized. There is a lower concentration of salivary Immunoglobulin A (IgA) in affected animals when compared with healthy cats. Thus, pain, anorexia, halitosis, weight loss and dehydration are common clinical manifestations in this important oral disease. To date there is no effective treatment. Because of its chronicity, the therapy should be individualized, aiming to minimize contact with oral bacterial antigens. Periodontal disease has no cure, only control. It presents as inflammation of the gums (gingivitis) and destruction of supporting tissues of the teeth (periodontitis), caused by the presence of biofilm. Treatment consists in removal of dental calculus and maintaining proper oral hygiene. Feline tooth resorption is an irreversible and extremely painful disease of unknown etiology. Clinical alterations are lesions of the enamel and / or cementum associated with severe gingivitis, usually on the tooth neck region. The most affected teeth are premolars and canines. Treatment involves dental extraction. It may be associated with periodontal disease. Teeth with pulp necrosis are a potent source of antigenic periapical destruction of parenchyma. Fractured canine tooth with pulp exposure requires a specific approach with endodontic therapy. The successful diagnosis and treatment of major oral diseases in cats depends on deep dental knowledge as well as the feline behavior.

INTRODUCTION

Despite often being neglected, disorders of the oral cavity are a constant in feline medicine, the second most frequent alteration in domestic cats, second only to musculoskeletal disorders and may be responsible for mood swings to systemic involvement once that cats are experts at hiding pain.

These conditions may also present worsened if associated with systemic viral infections such as feline immunodeficiency viral (FIV), Feline Viral Leukemia (FeLV), Calicivirose (FCV) and Feline Herpesvirus (FHV-1). Among oral diseases relevant to felines, the most common in clinical routine felines are chronic gingivostomatitis, periodontal disease, tooth resorption and chronic periapical lesion by the canine tooth fracture.

Clinical signs such as loss of appetite, lethargy, drooling and even aggression, which reflect discomfort and pain, may culminate in dehydration and loss of body condition with irreversible and even fatal systemic consequences.

In cats, as in other domestic animals, exposure to antigens of oral mucosa is a constant, but the physiological balance between these antigens and the immune system ensures the state of oral health. The main diseases of the oral cavity in domestic cats result from the imbalance of this important relationship, the loss of which can trigger an inappropriate inflammatory response - insufficient or exacerbated, especially if the patient is a carrier of feline systemic viral infection.

Dentition of the Domestic Cat

The knowledge of the main features of the dentition of domestic cats as knowledge of their dental formula and chronology of eruption, are of great importance in the evaluation, diagnosis and treatment planning of oral diseases of domestic cats.

Dental formula:

- Deciduous dentition: 2 x (i 3/3, 1/1 c, p 3/2) * = 26
- Permanent Dentition: 2 x (3/3 I, C 1/1, P 3/2, M 1/1) * = 30

* i and I - incisors; c and C - canine teeth; p e P - premolars and M teeth - molars.

*Lowercase letters indicate primary teeth and permanent teeth caps.

The domestic feline lacks the second pre molars or first and second pre molars; first molar is absent in most cases.

The chronology of tooth eruption of domestic cats is of great value in clinical practice, especially in the examination of the oral cavity. The dental formula of the domestic cat also applies to other felines. The chronology of tooth eruption is as follows:

- Deciduous incisors: 2 -3semanas
- Permanent Incisors: 3-4 months
- Deciduous canines: 3-4 weeks
- Permanent Canines: 4-5 months
- Pre molars: 3-6 weeks
- Pre Molars: 4-6 months
- Deciduous molars: absent
- Permanent Molars: 4-5 months

Feline Chronic Gingivostomatitis

Without certain cause, prevalence by gender or race, it can often affects animals aged from eight years. No definitive treatment is also known as linfoplasmocytic stomatitis, chronic ulcerative stomatitis, chronic gingivitis, plasma cell gingivofaringitis.

This important feline oral disease is characterized by proliferative ulcerative lesions, resulting from focal or diffuses inflammatory response mainly in the oral mucosa region glossopalatine, buccal mucosa, gingiva and alveolar mucosa. Because it is a disease with immune involvement, it responds more intensely in the presence of local and systemic diseases of bacterial and viral origin. Thus, the feline immunodeficiency virus (FIV), feline leukemia virus (FeLV) and calicivirose (FCV) contribute to periodontal disease exacerbation of the disease.

Antibody production occurs as a chronic immunological response to the prevalence of gum disease with lymphocytes and plasma cells that are the predominant immunoglobulin in such chronic disease. The complement system is activated by antibodies produced by plasma cells, which also cause injury to the cells of the stratified squamous epithelium of the gingiva; Local vascular permeability increases and severe gingival retraction occurs.

The most common clinical signs are halitosis, decreased appetite, drooling, dysphagia, weight loss and dehydration.

A detailed history and physical examination of the oral cavity preferably with the aid of chemical restraint (due to severe pain), as well observation of clinical signs are sufficient to do the diagnosis. However, additional diagnostic laboratory tests such as blood count, biochemistry and biopsy of inflammatory lesions should be performed. Tests for feline immunodeficiency virus, feline leukemia virus and calicivirosis are also indicated. The pain management is essential throughout follow-up.

As yet there is no definitive treatment therapy should be specific for each patient seeking to provide reduction of oral pain by reducing contact with oral antigens. The surgical approach through complete periodontal treatment with removal of teeth with periodontal involvement or removal of all premolar and molar teeth in severe cases associated with the clinical approach with systemic antibiotic therapy administering amoxicillin plus clavulanic acid has been satisfactory in 80% of cases.

The dedication of the owner is an important therapeutic pillar and, for this reason, it is crucial that it be properly informed by the complexity of the disease and the risk of failure in therapy.

Periodontal Disease

Periodontal disease is one of the problems identified in the oral cavity of cats. This disease has no cure, only control. Due to dental anatomy and inflammatory response characteristics of cats, its evolution requires a particular monitoring.

Periodontal disease is presented initially restricted to the periodontum as protective compound the gingiva (gingivitis) and subsequently inflammation as a result of untreated gingivitis, destruction of periodontal support composed of the periodontal ligament and alveolar bone, cementum (periodontitis) occurs. The primary cause of this condition is the presence of biofilm or plaque accumulated supra and sub gingival.

Gingivitis is clinically observed as edema, hyperemia and bleeding, and may present as a generalized or localized form.

In periodontitis there is a loss of the structures responsible for dental static: receding gums, resorption of alveolar bone and cementum exposure, culminating in tooth mobility and subsequent tooth loss. Halitosis is constant. It is an extremely painful process. Due to its microbiological characteristics, it is commonly associated with chronic gingivostomatitis in the domestic cats.

The diagnosis is determined based on history, clinical periodontal assessment and through intra-oral or preferably periapical radiographs, which allow the correct evaluation of the alveolar bone of all teeth.

The main goals of treatment of periodontal disease are to control the infection and restore the periodontal tissue and tissue health. It is composed of active periodontal therapy and periodontal supportive therapy. The basic active periodontal therapy accomplishes the removal of dental calculus, plaque and extraction of elements with the mobility ending with the crown polishing. The periodontal supportive therapy aims to preserve the results of active periodontal therapy, decreasing the recurrence of periodontal disease. The higher the formation of dental plaque, the greater will be the toxin produced in the gingival sulcus. The result of this process is to increase the intensity of inflammation and capillary permeability which cause increased flow of gingival exudate and contribute to the development of the periodontal pathogens. To help control periodontopathogenic microorganisms and the favorable immune response, systemic antibiotic therapy is an important therapeutic arsenal because it hit structures as furcations, mucous tubules and tonsils. The most commonly used drugs in these cases are amoxicillin (associated or not with clavulanic acid), lincosamides, quinolones and metronidazole. Mechanical control with toothbrushing is not usually feasible for most owners of cats. Thus, the effective control of bacterial plaque or biofilm and inflammation is the basis of control and treatment of periodontal diseases.

Feline Tooth Resorption

The resorption is critical in the root resorption process (physiological root resorption) of deciduous teeth for their exfoliation and eruption of permanent teeth. However, feline tooth resorption is pathological with high incidence. It is an irreversible and extremely painful disease, with prevalence in animals aged less than five years. The most affected teeth by this disease are the premolars although other teeth may also be affected by this disease.

In response to this resorptive process, severe gingivitis and gingival hyperplasia can be observed that the surface being affected by erosive lesions may be covered by gingival epithelium affected. Tooth loss is commonly associated with severe gingivitis.

Clinically, the most frequent signs are halitosis, gingivitis and gingival hyperplasia related to the affected tooth, dental erosive lesions commonly related to dental cervix, signs of pain during feeding, dysphagia and consequent anorexia and appetite loss.

Diagnosis is based on history, clinical signs and detailed clinical examination of the oral cavity, preferably with the patient under chemical restraint. The radiographic intraoral approach is essential for an accurate assessment and an early and differential diagnosis.

The origin and degree of involvement determine the stages of the disease, ranging from the metabolism of enamel or cementum to the total loss of tooth structure. For treatment plan is critical to determine the degree of injury. However, surgical therapy for extraction of all affected elements is the most successful, despite requiring professional knowledge of the field of instrumental and surgical maneuvers for its execution safely, because in many cases there may be root fragments, so sclerotic roots as crowns weakened by the erosive characteristics of this process. Restorative dental therapy is not justified since the process is progressive and irreversible. Treatment involves monitoring clinical and radiographic lesions until extraction, which does not rule out the importance and necessity of postoperative radiographic control inherent in the technique.

Dental Fracture

Fractured teeth with pulp necrosis are a potent source of antigenic sponsor periapical destruction of parenchyma and sometimes determining exacerbations. Dental fracture with and without frequent pulp exposure in cats requires a specific approach and need to prevent the spread of odontogenic infection there may be infiltration through the dentinal tubules exposed even in small fractures of the canine tooth. As the pulp is imprisoned by the dentinal wall is inelastic edema, inflammation progresses to necrosis. The odontogenic infection can also extend to surrounding tissues and reach the face.

According to the affected structures and the location of the tooth fracture the classification is established.

The most common causes of tooth fracture are related to behavioral peculiarities of felines (fighting for females or territories), falls by any known ("paratrooper cat syndrome"), characteristics of dental anatomy (the canine teeth of cats are longer and thin - mostly upper canines) and hit by a car. Therefore, special attention should be devoted to evaluating patients unsterilized. The feline oral cavity is visible in only 30% to the human eye in domestic conditions. For this reason, commonly the owner does not observe the fractured tooth and when it does, the periapical lesion is already installed because the pulp responds with inflammation leading to edema.

Diagnosis is therefore made based on history, clinical and radiographic oral examination. Root canal therapy is indicated as an alternative to tooth extraction when the line of tooth fractures and does not compromise the integrity of the stomatognathic system.

The successful diagnosis and treatment of major oral diseases in cats depends on deep knowledge of odonto-stomatological and dental materials and techniques to use as well as the domain of the peculiarities of the behavior of the domestic cat and his owner.

REFERENCES

Chardieu, G. E. Blaizot, A. Gingivites et stomatites félines. *Pratique édicale et Chirurgicale de l'Animal de Compagn*ie, 1999, 34, 135-144.

Harvey, C. E. Oral inflammatory diseases in cats. *Journal of American Hospital Association,* 1991, v.27, p.585-591.

Hennet, P. Relationship between oral calicivirus and herpesvirus carriage and "palatoglossitis" lesions. In: Annual Veterinary Dental Forum & World Veterinary Dental Congress Ix, 2005, Orlando. Proceedings…Orlando: Academy of Veterinary Dentistry, American Veterinary Dental College, *American Veterinary Dental Society*, p.503, 2005.

Lommer, M. J.; Verstraete, F. J. M. Concurrent oral shedding of feline calicivirus and herpervirus 1 in cats with chronic gingivostomatitis. *Oral Microbiology and Immunology*, San Francisco, 2003, v.18, p.131-134.

Pedersen, N. C. Inflamatory oral cavity diseases of the cat. *Veterinary Clinic North America Small Animal Practioner*, 1992, v.22, n.6, p.1323-1345.

Reiter, A. M.; Lewis, J. R.; Okuda, A. Update on the Etiology of Tooth resorption in domestic cats. In: Dentistry – The veterinary clinics of North

America – Small Animal Practice. W. B. Sounders Company, 2005, vol. 35, n. 4, p.913-942.

Rochette, J. Treating the inflammed mouth. *Congress World Small Animal Veterinary Association,* Vancouver, Canada. 2001.

Rose, L. R.; Mealey, B. L.; Genco, R.J.; Cohen, D.W.; Periodontia-medicina, ciruurgia e implantes, Editora Santos, 2007.

Roza, M. R. Odontologia em pequenos animais. Rio de Janeiro: *L. F. Livros de Veterinária,* 2004.

Wiggs, R. B.; Lobprise, H. B. Veterinary Dentistry: principles and practice. *Lippincott-Raven*, 1997.

In: Felines
Editor: Colleen Kevins

ISBN: 978-1-63463-550-9

Chapter 5

MELATONIN AS A NEW THERAPEUTIC STRATEGY FOR FELINE UVEITIS TREATMENT

María José Del Sole[1], Ruth E. Rosenstein[2,*] and Pablo H. Sande[2]

[1]Small Animal Teaching Hospital, Clinic Department, School of Veterinary Science, National University of the Center of Buenos Aires Province, Tandil, CIVETAN/CONICET, Buenos Aires Province, Argentina.

[2]Laboratory of Retinal Neurochemistry and Experimental Ophthalmology, Department of Human Biochemistry, School of Medicine/CEFyBO, University of Buenos Aires/CONICET, Buenos Aires, Argentina

ABSTRACT

Uveitis is the most common form of intraocular inflammation and a disease with potentially blinding sequels. Since the disease causes significant morbidity and the use of traditional forms of treatment is restricted by limited effectiveness and considerable side effects, uveitis remains a challenging field to veterinary ophthalmologists. Current

---

* Corresponding author: Department of Human Biochemistry, School of Medicine, CEFyBO, University of Buenos Aires, CONICET, Paraguay 2155, 5th floor, (1121), Buenos Aires, ARGENTINA, Tel: 54-11-45083672 (ext 37), Fax: 54-11-45083672 (ext 31), Email: ruthr@fmed.uba.ar.

understanding of the role of oxidative and nitrosative stress in ocular inflammatory diseases indicates that antioxidant and antinitridergic therapy may be important to optimize the uveitis treatment. Several lines of evidence strongly support that melatonin is a potent antioxidant molecule which is effective in scavenging free radicals that are generated in ocular tissues, and it inhibits the retinal nitridergic pathway. In view of the fact that melatonin lacks significant adverse collateral effects even at high doses, melatonin could potentially protect ocular tissues by effectively scavenging free radicals and excessive amounts of NO generated in the uveitic eye. This chapter summarizes recent investigations showing that melatonin prevents clinical, biochemical, ultrastructural and functional consequences of experimental uveitis, and which support the role of melatonin as a therapeutic strategy for uveitis treatment.

Keywords: Melatonin, uveitis, nitric oxide, oxidative damage, feline uveitis

Abbreviations

AA: arachidonic acid
AH: aqueous humor
BOB: blood-ocular barrier
BAB: blood-aqueous barrier
BRB: blood-retinal barrier
COX: cyclooxygenase
EIU: endotoxin induced uveitis
ERG: electroretinogram
FeLV: feline leukemia virus
FIP: feline infectious peritonitis
iNOS: inducible isoform of NO synthase
IOP: intraocular pressure
LIU: lens-induced uveitis
LPS: bacterial lipopolysaccharide
NOS: NO synthase
NSAIDs: nonsteroidal anti-inflammatory drugs
PGs: prostaglandins
ROS: reactive oxygen species
RPE: retinal pigment epithelium
TNF-α: tumor necrosis factor α.

FELINE UVEITIS

The term uveitis refers to the inflammation of the middle vascular (uveal) tunic of the eye, localized between the outer fibrous (corneoescleral) tunic and the inner neurosensory (retinal) tunic and involves the uveal tissues (iris, ciliary body, and choroid) and adjacent ocular structures (retina, vitreous, and optic nerve). Depending on the structures involved in the inflammatory process, uveitis is classified as anterior, intermediate, and posterior uveitis. In anterior uveitis, the iris (iritis) and/or the anterior part of the ciliary body (iridocyclitis) are affected; intermediate uveitis affects the posterior part of the ciliary body (*pars planitis*) and anterior choroid, while posterior uveitis primarily involves the choroid (choroiditis), although due to its proximity to the retina, the inflammation of both structures (retinochoroiditis or chorioretinitis) is frequent (Wilkie, 1994; Collins and Moore, 1999; Barnett and Crispin, 2000, Maggs, 2009). The term panuveitis denotes inflammation of the choroid, iris, and ciliary body. Although these anatomic divisions are useful, inciting antigens, effector cells, and cytokines rarely are restricted to one compartment alone, and pure anterior or posterior uveitis should never be assumed as such (Wilkie, 1994; Collins and Moore, 1999; Barnett and Crispin, 2000; Maggs 2009). The posterior segment involvement may decrease the probability of maintaining a healthy ocular globe, and in this case, therapeutic agents should be systemically administered.

CAUSES OF UVEITIS IN CATS

Although uveitis in cats may be provoked by corneal ulceration, penetrating wound, or blunt trauma, infectious systemic diseases are the most frequent causes, particularly due to the highly vascular nature and the immunosensibility of the uveal tract. The causes of uveitis are diverse and frequently elusive. Even after a very complete diagnostic testing, the cause is not elucidated in as many as 70% of cats with uveitis (Davidson et al., 1991). According to Davidson et al. (1991), the most commonly identified agents are feline leukemia virus (FeLV) and the most commonly identified cause of uveitis was lymphosarcoma or melanoma. In another study including 139 cats (158 globes), a cause was identified only in 67% of cases, and the most common diagnoses were feline infectious peritonitis (FIP), FeLV-associated lymphosarcoma, and trauma (Peiffer and Wilcock, 1991). In that context, although feline uveitis can be classified as infectious, inflammatory, traumatic and neoplastic, the most clinically relevant classifications are a two-category systems: on one hand, uveitis can be categorized as idiopathic or having an identified cause, and on the other hand, uveitis could be attributed to endogenous or exogenous causes (Powell and Lappin, 2001). Examples of exogenous causes include trauma, lens luxation, and ulcerative keratitis, the last produces a so-called 'reflex uveitis' via stimulation of the trigeminal nerve. Exogenous causes are usually more obvious and tend to be associated with other ocular signs which can be identified after a thorough ophthalmic examination. In cats, endogenous causes are more frequent, produce more subtle clinical signs, require more diagnostic verification, and are more resistant to treatment than exogenous causes.

According to several reports, approximately 30% to 62% of affected cats had no identifiable concurrent systemic disease (Gemensky et al., 1996; Chavkin et al., 1992). Feline immunodeficiency virus (FIV), FIP, FeLV, *Toxoplasma gondii*, *Cryptococcus neoformans*, and *Histoplasma capsulatum* are the most frequent infectious agents implicated in the disease (Peiffer and Wilcock, 1991; Lappin et al., 1992; Glaze and Gelatt, 1999; Barnett and Crispin, 2000; Lappin, 2000). However, *Blastomyces dermatitidis, Coccidioides immitis and Candida albicans* (Lappin et al., 1992; Glaze and Gelatt, 1999; Barnett and Crispin, 2000; Lappin, 2000), *Bartonella henselae* (Lappin et al., 1999), *Borrelia burgdorferi* (Magnarelli et al, 2005), feline herpes virus 1 (FHV 1) (Lappin, 2000), *Ehrlichia canis* (Breitschwerdt et al, 2002), *Leishmania* spp. (Leiva et al, 2005; Verneuil, 2013; Richter et al, 2014), *Cuterebra* spp. (Johnson et al., 1988; Harris et al., 2000), *Mycobacterium bovis, Mycobacterium tuberculosis* and *Mycobacterium avium* (Gunn-Moore et al., 1996), and *Metastrongylidae* (Glaze and Gelatt, 1999) were also associated with feline uveitis (Table 1).

Clinical Manifestations

In general terms, uveitis starts with a local lesion of the blood-ocular barrier (BOB) (Barnett and Crispin, 2000). The acute response to uveal damage is a brief vasoconstriction followed by a prolonged dilation of the arteriola-capilar-venule unit, which leads to an alteration of the vascular permeability. Although all the iridal vasculature has the same endothelial intercellular junctions (Glaze and Gelatt, 1999), feline iridal capillaries have discontinuous endothelial cells (Bellhorn, 1980) which favour the development of uveitis in this species. Therefore, proteins, erythrocytes (hyphema) and leukocytes (hypopyon) leave the vascular lumen and accumulate into the aqueous humour (AH), provoking anterior chamber turbidity (Tyndall effect). In addition, proteins and pigments from macrophages and pigmented stromal cells of the iris (Collins and Moore, 1999) can focally accumulate on the corneal endothelium (keratic precipitates), gravitate in the ventral anterior chamber (hypopyon) or infiltrate in the hypervascularised iris (rubeosis iridis), generating iridal swelling (Barnett and Crispin, 2000). Moreover, if the initial bleeding is extensive or continuous, red blood cell complete filling of the anterior chamber can occur (Glaze and Gelatt, 1999). The intraocular inflammation could also provoke hyperemia in anterior ciliary and conjunctivae vessels (Glaze and Gelatt, 1999; Barnett and Crispin, 2000). Acute inflammation of the anterior uvea provokes pain, manifested by blepharospasm, photophobia, excessive tearing, and retraction of the eyeball (enophthalmos), with passive or active protrusion of the third eyelid (Barnett and Crispin, 2000). However, intraocular pain is difficult to interpret in animals, especially cats. They seem far more likely to show subtle and less localizing signs such as lethargy, anorexia, or reduced interaction with their owner or environment (Maggs 2009).

The decrease of intraocular pressure (IOP) as a consequence of a reduction in AH production provoked by cyclitis (Barnett and Crispin, 2000), or an increase in the uveoescleral flow mediated by prostaglandins (PGs) (Glaze and Gelatt, 1999), is an early indicator of uveitis (Glaze and Gelatt, 1999), and thus, tonometry is one of the most sensitive tests for monitoring uveitis during treatment (Maggs 2010). In chronic processes, ciliary body fibrosis, atrophy, or both contribute to the decrease of the secretor function and eye hypotony (Glaze and Gelatt, 1999). We have demonstrated consistent daily variations of IOP in cats exposed to a light-dark cycle, with maximal values during the night (Del Sole et al., 2007). In this report, we showed that nocturnal IOP values in some uveitic animals were close to diurnal IOP in healthy eyes suggesting that the assessment of daily variations of IOP could contribute to a better uveitis diagnosis in felines (Del Sole et al., 2007).

Pupillary constriction or miosis is induced by PGs and other inflammatory mediators, by direct action on the sphincter muscle. However, anterior or posterior synechiae kept contracted or moderately dilated pupils, which result in a fixed or deformed pupil (Glaze and Gelatt, 1999).

Table 1. Most frequent causes of feline uveitis

Exogenous	Endogenous
Trauma	Infectious
Penetrating wound	Feline immunodeficiency virus (FIV)
Blunt trauma	Feline leukemia virus (FeLV)
Reflex uveitis	Feline infectious peritonitis (FIP)
Lens luxation	Feline herpesvirus 1 (FHV 1)
	Cryptococcus neoformans
	Histoplasma capsulatum
	Coccidioides immitis
	Blastomyces dermatitidis
	Candida albicans
	Aspergillus spp.
	Fungi dematiáceos
	Bartonella spp.
	Micobacteryum spp.
	Ehrlichia spp.
	Borrelia burgdorferi
	Parasitic
	Toxoplasma gondii
	Leishmania spp.
	Ophthalmomyiasis Cuterebra spp.
	Lens-induced uveitis (LIU)
	Idiopathic
	Neoplastic
	Diffuse iridial melanoma
	Primary ocular sarcomas
	Primary ciliary body adenomas and adenocarcinomas
	Lymphosarcoma (with or without associated FeLV or FIV)
	Metastatic uveal neoplasms (mainly adenocarcinoma)

Corneal edema observed in some cases, is a consequence of corneal endothelial cell dysfunction induced by inflammatory mediators in the AH (Collins and Moore, 1999). These cells are involved in maintaining a low concentration of water in the cornea through a Na^{+}-K^{+}/ATPase pump (Gum et al., 1999). In chronic cases, edema is caused by the leakage of fluid from deep perilimbal anterior ciliary vessels that invade the cornea towards the stroma (Barnett and Crispin, 2000). In cats, edema can be very subtle as compared with dogs (Maggs, 2009).

Active chorioretinitis is characterized by cell infiltration and edema, observed in the ophthalmoscopic examination as grayish foci. The blood-retinal barrier (BRB) alteration produces edema and retinal detachment, perivascular cuffing, and bleeding. In the inactive chorioretinitis, ophthalmic signs are: alteration of tapetal coloration, hyperpigmentation or hypopigmentation of the retinal pigment epithelium (RPE) and tapetal hyperreflectivity due to retinal thinning (Barnett and Crispin, 2000).

Except in lens-induced (LIU) and neoplastic uveitis, there are no specific ophthalmologic changes, particularly when the anterior uveal tract is affected (Lappin et al., 1992). However, some signs are frequently associated with some causes (Glaze and Gelatt, 1999). Mutton fat keratic precipitates occur most frequently in FIP and FeLV uveitis, while signs caused by FIP include haemorrhage (Glaze and Gelatt, 1999). FIV and FeLV uveitis are associated with iridal nodules, similarly to white to pink masses in anterior chamber or attached to the anterior portion of the iris in uveitis associated with FeLV (Glaze and Gelatt, 1999). Infiltrated cells in anterior vitreous and formation of synechiae, as well as cortical cataracts, and glaucoma occur more frequently with uveitis associated to FIV (Glaze and Gelatt, 1999). FIP involves panuveitis or panophthalmitis with vitritis, chorioretinitis, marked anterior uveitis, severe and diffuse corneal edema and inflammatory retinal detachments (Glaze and Gelatt, 1999). In addition, anterior uveitis provoked by FeLV can progress to a diffuse inflammation of the eyeball or a tumour formation (Glaze and Gelatt, 1999).

Ophthalmic Complications

Complications associated to anterior or posterior uveitis are directly related to the duration and causes of the uveal inflammation (Glaze and Gelatt, 1999). Anterior synechiae occur if the iris is adhered to the corneal endothelium. If they are extensive, posterior synechiae may occlude the AH flow from the posterior chamber through the pupil into the anterior chamber, causing iris bombe (anterior ballooning of the iris), and secondary glaucoma (Cassin and Rubin, 2001). Preiridal fibrovascular membranes may be formed on the anterior surface of the iris. Clinically, the term rubeosis iridis is applied, because the neovascular membrane on the anterior iridal surface causes a reddish cast to the iris (Cassin and Rubin, 2001).

Chronic inflammation often induces cataracts, presumably by the diffusion of inflammatory mediators across the lens capsule, causing lens epithelial metaplasia, necrosis, or posterior migration, as well as lens fiber degeneration, liquefaction, and necrosis (Eagle and Spencer, 1996; Streeten, 2000).

Although lens luxation seems to be relatively rare in dogs (Curtis et al., 1983), chronic uveitis is a frequent cause of lens luxation in cats, because zonular fibers can be degraded by inflammatory products in the AH (Olivero et al., 1991). Secondary glaucoma may occur due to pupillary block as a result of iris bombe or lens luxation or may be attributable to occlusion of the iridocorneal angle by peripheral anterior synechiae (Stiles and Towsend, 2007). The final consequence of the inflammatory process could be buphtalmus or eyeball atrophy (*pthisis bulbis*) (Glaze and Gelatt, 1999).

CHEMICAL MEDIATORS OF INFLAMMATION

Despite that uveitis is one of the main causes of eye morbidity and loss of visual functions, the complexity of the biochemical and immune mechanisms involved in its generation and development remain incompletely elucidated. Several lines of evidence support that uveitis is due to damage generated by infiltrated leukocytes which release cytokines (de Vos et al., 1994; Planck et al., 1994), and other inflammatory chemical mediators, like arachidonic acid (AA) metabolites (Bellot et al., 1996), reactive oxygen species (ROS) (Rao, 1990), NO (Hashida et al., 2000), and superoxide anion (O_2^-) (Jacquemin et al., 1996), among many others. Oxygen-derived free radicals have been implicated in the inflammation associated with endotoxin-induced uveitis (EIU) (Satici et al., 2003). Free radicals initiate retinal lipid peroxidation, and the resultant hydroperoxides serve as amplification factors, such as chemotaxis of inflammatory cells (Goto et al., 1991; Wu et al., 1992). Oxidative stress in photoreceptor mitochondria appears to be an early event in the development of uveitis, which initiates the subsequent irreversible retinal damage by attracting phagocytic cells to the initial site of injury (Saraswathy and Rao, 2008). In fact, there is evidence that free radical scavengers and antioxidants can act as anti-inflammatory agents, protecting the eye from inflammation-mediated tissue damage (Bosch-Morell et al., 2002).

NO is a highly reactive short-lived radical species which plays an important role as an intern and intracellular messenger in the central nervous system. NO is generated by a family of enzymes called NOS that oxidate L-arginine to L-citrulline producing NO. NO acts as an endogenous activator of a soluble guanylyl cyclase, and thereby it increases cGMP levels. In the retina as in other tissues, NO can be neuroprotective and neurodestructive, depending on the redox state and on its concentration (Kashiwagi et al., 2001). NO can react with superoxide producing peroxynitrite, a powerful and deleterious oxidant which triggers apoptotic cell death (Sennlaub et al., 2002). In a model of oxygen-induced retinopathy, it was demonstrated that iNOS is upregulated in response to tissue ischemia, is cytotoxic and inhibits vascular repair (Stevenson et al., 2010). In addition, a significant activation of the retinal nitridergic pathway was observed in hypertensive eyes (Belforte et al., 2007). Parks et al. (1994) demonstrated that multiple intraperitoneal injections of N-omega-nitro-L-arginine methyl ester (L-NAME), a well-known NO synthase (NOS) inhibitor, reduced clinical signs of EIU, suggesting that NO could participate in the pathogenesis of experimental uveitis as a proinflammatory mediator. Furthermore, it has been shown that hemodynamic and vascular permeability changes associated with EIU in rats are in part due to the increased production of NO. High levels of nitrite in the AH and vitreous of rats at the time of maximal ocular inflammation following bacterial lipopolysaccharide (LPS) injection, and the presence of a calcium independent NOS activity in the anterior segment during EIU (Mandai et al., 1994) have been demonstrated. In addition, reverse transcriptase-PCR assays show an increased expression of the inducible isoform of NOS (iNOS) mRNA in the iris-ciliary body and in the retina of rats with experimental uveitis (Goureau et al., 1995). *In situ* hybridization revealed that epithelial cells of the iris-ciliary body and cells infiltrating (macrophages, polymorphonuclear leukocytes) the anterior segment and the retina are the major source of NO (Jacquemin et al., 1996). Moreover, a significant correlation between nitrite levels in the AH and clinical signs of EIU was observed. The efficacy of treatment with NOS inhibitors in EIU in rats or rabbits suggests that treatments that reduce NO production or NO action would be beneficial and would provide new prospects for uveitis treatment (Becquet et al., 1997).

Prostaglandins (PGs) can be synthesized through the activities of two cyclooxygenase (COX) isoforms. COX-1 is constitutively expressed in most tissues and its activity provides for the relatively small amounts of PGs required for the mediation and modulation of normal physiological functions. In inflammatory conditions, COX-2 is rapidly induced by cytokines, growth factors, and LPS, and its enzymatic activity accounts for the large amounts of PGs produced during inflammation (Masferrer and Kulkarni, 1997). Small doses of PGs topically or intraocularly administered reproduce some of inflammatory signs, such as hyperaemia, miosis, breakdown of the blood-aqueous barrier (BAB) and ocular hypertension. In addition, PGE_2 topically administered together with histamine (but not each one of these compounds alone) cause cellular infiltration and produce edema in conjunctival tissues (Bhattacherjee, 1980). Moreover, it was shown that AA metabolites regulate vascular permeability, chemotaxis, and contribute to uveitis amplification (Bhattacherjee, 1980; Howes and McKay, 1976).

Current Therapy for Feline Uveitis

The best treatment relies on the identification and removal or reduction of the causative antigen; however, this is rarely possible. An early diagnosis and a rapidly and completely controlled intraocular inflammation are critical factors, due to the close anatomical relationship of the uvea with components directly implicated in visual functions. Thus, immunomodulatory drugs are the mainstay of uveitis therapy (Maggs, 2009). Topical mydriatics, topical (and, in select cases, systemic) corticosteroids, and nonsteroidal anti-inflammatory drugs (NSAIDs) are agents frequently used to attain those goals. In addition, parasympatholytic drugs have multiple favourable actions in uveitic eyes, because these drugs paralyze the parasympathetically innervated iris sphincter and ciliary body muscles, causing mydriasis and cycloplegia, respectively (Klauss and Constantinescu, 2004). The most often used mydriatic agent is atropine (1%) ointment or solution. The use of the ointment is indicated in felines, because the bitter taste of atropine solution may provoke particularly marked reactions in cats (Gelatt et al., 1973). The pupillary dilation reduces leakage of vascular elements into the AH by causing radial blood vessels within the iris stroma to 'concertina', decreases the iris surface area (from which inflammatory mediators and vascular components originate), reduces uveal vascular endothelial permeability, and in turn decreases the risks and consequences of posterior synechiae. However, 'bunching' of the iris in the periphery does increase the risk of anterior synechiae and potentially obstruction of the iridocorneal angle. In these patients, the effect of mydriasis on IOP can be tested by a single application of the short acting drug tropicamide, followed by tonometry when the pupil is fully dilated. If IOP is increased by tropicamide, atropine should not be administered (Maggs, 2009). Atropine should be applied to effect and it should still be administered to patients with synechiae since the analgesia resulting from cycloplegia should not be affected (Maggs 2009). An alternative cycloplegic medication, if a risk of secondary glaucoma exists, is tropicamide. Tropicamide is a short acting parasympatholytic that typically lasts 4 to 6 hours and can be discontinued if IOP becomes elevated (Colitz, 2005).

Corticosteroids are frequently used to suppress inflammation (Holmberg and Maggs, 2004). To control anterior uveitis, topical application is often the preferred route because it allows for high local drug concentrations, reducing systemic side effects (Holmberg and Maggs, 2004). Prednisolone acetate (1%) ophthalmic suspension, and dexamethasone (0.1%) are able to penetrate an intact corneal epithelium (Wilkie, 1990). Therefore, systemic therapy is imperative for posterior uveitis. The use of glucocorticoids, such as prednisone, prednisolone, or dexamethasone to suppress inflammation within the posterior segment (chorioretinitis) requires a systemic administration or, occasionally, immunosuppressive doses (Holmberg and Maggs, 2004).

NSAIDs can be particularly useful in cases of mild anterior uveitis, as adjunctive therapy when combined with topical corticosteroids, and to control posterior segment inflammation when an infectious aetiology cannot be completely discarded, or until lymphosarcoma is eliminated as a differential diagnosis. They may be preferred in patients with diabetes or other endocrinopathies in which corticosteroid use may not be recommended. NSAIDs block the synthesis of PGs (Giuliano, 2004), suppress polymorphonuclear cell locomotion and chemotaxis (Perianin et al., 1985), decrease expression of inflammatory cytokines (Leonardi et al., 2000), and may act as free radical scavengers (Flach, 1992). However, only a few NSAIDs have been evaluated regarding their efficacy in controlling ocular inflammation. Flunixin meglumine and aspirin have been shown to stabilize the BAB in experimental models of uveitis (Millichamp et al., 1991; Ward et al., 1992); flunixin meglumine had good effects, whereas the effects of aspirin are moderate when compared with placebo. The relative efficacies have been studied in an anterior chamber paracentesis model of uveitis in dogs, and the order of BAB stabilizing efficacy was as follows: diclofenac > flurbiprofen > suprofen > tolmetin which was similar to placebo (Ward, 1996).

Despite the beneficial effects, the immunosuppressive effect of corticoids may contribute to the development of the systemic disease and their chronic use could induce cortisonic glaucoma (Zhan et al., 1992), while NSAIDs may delay the reparation process and coagulation, provoke acute renal insufficiency, gastrointestinal haemorrhage or ulceration (Wilkie, 1994; Barnett and Crispin, 2000), and have the risk of bone marrow suppression and haemorrhage in cats (Powell and Lappin, 2001). In addition, NSAIDs are not immunosuppressive, and in some countries are more expensive, sold in smaller volumes and may not be available in ointment form. Moreover, it has been shown that only 33% of animals with uveitis associated with systemic diseases respond to this treatment (Gemensky et al., 1996). There are several common features for uveitis among different species. However, many antiuveitic medications that are successfully used in humans and dogs are not very well tolerated by cats and, therefore, the selection of recommended drugs is limited in this species. Acquiring this knowledge relies heavily on the use of experimental models particularly developed in this species.

EXPERIMENTAL MODELS OF FELINE UVEITIS

An experimental model of feline uveitis would greatly facilitate the understanding of the cellular events involved in ocular inflammation as well as the development of new therapeutic strategies for uveitis in cats. In that context, ocular toxoplasmosis in cats was experimentally induced *via* inoculation of a low number of organisms from a mildly virulent strain of *Toxoplasma gondii* into the common carotid artery (Davidson, 1993). However, the pathogenicity of *Toxoplasma gondii* depends on the virulence of the strain, which could make difficult to reproduce the experimental model in different laboratories. Moreover, a mild inflammation in the anterior segment was observed following inoculation with *Toxoplasma gondii* in cats, whereas naturally occurring uveitis generally involves a more generalized ocular inflammation. Furthermore, experimentally induced ocular toxoplasmosis was associated with the breakdown of the retinal pigment epithelium cell barrier, whereas disruption of both anterior and posterior BOB should be modeled in order to more closely reproduce feline uveitis. Finally, ocular toxoplasmosis is a specific form of ocular disease, whereas an "ideal" experimental model of feline uveitis should reproduce pathological consequences caused by a greater variety of etiopathogenic agents.

Endotoxin-induced uveitis (EIU) is an animal model of acute ocular inflammation induced by administration of LPS, a component of Gram-negative bacterial outer membranes (Rosembuan et al., 1980; Forrester et al., 1980; Csukas et al., 1990). LPS enhances the expression of various inflammatory mediators, such as interleukin-6 (IL-6) (Hoekzema et al., 1991), tumor necrosis factor α (TNF-α) (Chi et al., 2004), PGE_2 (Rao et al., 1987) and monocyte chemotactic protein -1 (de Vos et al., 1994), as well as the production of NO (Rao 1990), which contribute to the inflammation process, resulting in the breakdown of the BOB and leukocyte infiltration. Although EIU was originally used as a model of anterior uveitis, increasing evidences show that it also involves inflammation of the posterior segment of the eye with recruitment of leukocytes that adhere to the retinal vasculature and infiltrate the vitreous cavity (Kurihara et al., 2006; Yomura et al., 2007, Sande et al., 2008). In this vein, we have developed an experimental model of EIU in cats (Del Sole et al., 2008). For this purpose, we used a unilateral intravitreal injection of LPS because this maneuver avoids the development of systemic inflammation and allows the use of the contralateral eye as a control, thereby decreasing the risk of treatment-related death, and minimizing the number of animals. The clinical consequences of LPS injection during a 45-day period were assessed by use of a scoring system and could be apportioned to approximately 3 phases: from days 1 through 12, from days 15 through 29, and from day 35 until the end of the study (day 45), respectively. In the first phase, most of the signs were observed in the anterior segment of LPS-injected eyes, whereas in the last phase, sequels in the posterior segment were most noticeable. Few studies of EIU in several species have previously addressed the temporal course of ocular alterations after LPS injection, and largely only short-term (from 24 hours to 7 days) consequences were reported. Our study indicates that a single intravitreal injection of LPS in cats induces ocular alterations compatible with feline uveitis, and that the duration of these effects is longer than previously estimated.

Regardless of the administration method used, the injection of LPS is known to provoke an increase in protein concentration and cell number in AH in rabbits, rats, and mice (Rosenbaum et al., 1980; Csukas et al., 1990; Kogiso et al., 1992). As expected, the intravitreal injection of LPS in cats provokes a significant increase in both parameters, supporting a disruption of the BOB integrity. In addition, a significant reduction in ERG a- and b-wave amplitude was detected in LPS-treated eyes, suggesting that sequels of ocular inflammation induced by LPS could affect the outer and middle retina. In agreement with this result, attenuation of the ERG a- and b-wave amplitude in various animals and even in humans with uveitis has been observed (Hamasaki et al., 1993; Kim et al., 1999; Horio et al., 2001). Moreover, at 45 days post-injection of LPS, retinal lesions, in particular inward foldings of photoreceptor external segments, and lymphocytes were observed in the inner region of the retina, indicating damage to the outer, middle, and inner retina. Moreover, similar to findings in cats with naturally occurring uveitis, IOP was significantly lower in LPS- than in vehicle-injected eyes. In summary, these results indicate that experimental uveitis induced by a single intravitreal injection of LPS in cats causes clinical, biochemical, histological, and functional alterations which are consistent with the main features of naturally occurring feline uveitis (Del Sole et al., 2008). Thus, this model may be a useful tool in the investigation of new treatment strategies for feline uveitis.

OCULAR FUNCTIONS OF MELATONIN

Melatonin is a ubiquitous natural substance widely distributed in nature, being found both in plants and animals (Hardeland and Poeggeler, 2003; Pandi-Perumal et al., 2006; Paredes et al., 2009). Although in all mammals including humans, melatonin is primarily synthesized in the pineal gland, its synthesis also occurs in various parts of the eye, i.e. the retina (Cardinali and Rosner, 1971a; 1971b; Faillace et al., 1995; Tosini and Menaker, 1998), the ciliary body (Martin et al., 1992) and the lachrymal gland (Mhatre et al., 1992).

Retinal melatonin acts as a neuromodulator that mediates dark adaptive regulation of retinomotor movements (Pierce and Besharse, 1985), and regulates dopamine release from amacrine cells. (Dubocovich, 1983). Both dopamine and melatonin are key signaling agents in the regulation of retinal rhythmicity. These two substances are mutually inhibitory, acting as signals for day and night, respectively. It was demonstrated that picomolar concentrations of melatonin selectively inhibit the calcium-dependent release of dopamine from rabbit retina (Dubocovich, 1983). The action of melatonin on the rod pathway at the level of horizontal and amacrine cells has been proposed as a unique mechanism by which the retina adapts to low light intensities (Scher et al., 2002). A correlation between melatonin levels and the electroretinographic response has been shown in humans which suggest that daily melatonin and electroretinogram (ERG) cycling are associated (Rufiange et al., 2002). On the other hand, melatonin decreases retinal cAMP accumulation (Faillace et al., 1994) and regulates the activity of the retinal glutamate/glutamine cycle activity (Sáenz et al., 2004).

MELATONIN AS A RETINAL ANTIOXIDANT

The possibility that melatonin could detoxify reactive oxygen species (ROS) was originally suggested by Ianas et al. (1991). Shortly thereafter, Poeggeler et al. (1993) and Reiter and coworkers (1994) using spin trapping and electron resonance spectroscopy, demonstrated melatonin's capacity to directly scavenge the highly reactive hydroxyl radical. Since then, several reports have shown that melatonin acts as a free radical scavenger and an efficient antioxidant (Hardeland et al., 1995; Reiter et al., 1997; 1998; 2000; Pandi-Perumal et al., 2006). Not only melatonin, but also several of its metabolites generated during its free radical scavenging action act as antioxidants (Tan et al., 2007). The kynurenic pathway of melatonin metabolism includes a series of radical scavengers with the possible sequence: Melatonin → cyclic 3-hydroxymelatonin → N^1-acetyl-N^2-formyl-5-methoxykynuramine (AFMK) → N^1-acetyl-5-methoxykynuramine. In the metabolic step from melatonin to AFMK, up to four free radicals can be consumed (Adler et al., 1997; Guenther et al., 2005; Hardeland, 2005; Tan et al., 2007). Because of this pathway, melatonin's efficacy as an antioxidant is greatly increased. Melatonin has been shown to protect against oxidative stress in various, highly divergent experimental systems. Melatonin's functions as an antioxidant include: a) direct free radical scavenging, b) stimulation of antioxidative enzymes, c) increasing the efficiency of mitochondrial oxidative phosphorylation and reducing electron leakage (thereby lowering free radical generation), and d) augmenting the efficiency of other antioxidants (Reiter et al., 2003). Melatonin has been shown to scavenge free radicals generated in mitochondria, reduce electron leakage from the respiratory complexes and improve ATP synthesis (Acuña-Castroviejo et al., 2003; Leon et al., 2005). Moreover, melatonin preserves mitochondrial glutathione levels, thereby enhancing the antioxidant potential (Leon et al., 2004).

The retina is particularly susceptible to oxidative stress because of its high consumption of oxygen, its high proportion of polyunsaturated fatty acids, and its direct exposure to light. It was demonstrated that melatonin decreases lipid peroxidation of polyunsaturated fatty acids located in rod outer segment membranes (Guajardo et al., 2003), it may protect retinal pigment epithelial cells from oxidative stress (Liang et al., 2004), and it prevents retinal oxidative damage from ischemia/reperfusion injury (Celebi et al., 2002). In cultures of human retinal neuronal cells subjected to experimental hypoxanthine/xanthine oxidase -induced injury, melatonin is able to rescue retinal neurons (Lee et al., 2001). Furthermore, in dark-adapted single photoreceptors isolated from the frog retina after illumination with saturating light, melatonin at picomolar and low nanomolar concentrations was shown to be 100 times more potent in inhibiting light-induced oxidative processes than vitamin E (Marchiafava and Longoni, 1999). Recently, we have shown that melatonin increases superoxide dismutase activity and reduced glutathione levels, whereas it decreases lipid peroxidation in the rat retina (Belforte et al., 2010). Taken together, these results strongly support the role of melatonin as an effective retinal antioxidant.

MELATONIN AND THE RETINAL NITRIDERGIC PATHWAY

In isolated conditions, melatonin may directly react with NO yielding at least one stable product, N-nitrosomelatonin, which was characterized by nuclear magnetic resonance (NMR) and X-ray spectroscopy (Turjanski et al., 2000a; 2000b). In addition to a direct scavenging of NO, low concentrations of melatonin significantly decrease hamster retinal NOS activity. Melatonin behaves as a non-competitive inhibitor of this enzyme, since it decreases the Vmax, with no changes on the Km (Sáenz et al., 2002). This result agrees with the previously described effect of melatonin on NOS from other neural structures such as hypothalamus (Bettahi et al., 1996), cerebellum (Pozo et al., 1997), striatum, and cerebral frontal cortex (León et al., 1998). However, while the inhibitory effect of melatonin in those tissues was evident up to 1 nM, a much higher sensitivity to the methoxyindole was evident in the retina, as it was effective even at 1 pM. In addition, while in other systems melatonin is active when added to crude homogenates, in the hamster retina, it is only effective when the whole tissues are preincubated in the presence of the methoxyindole. The high sensitivity of this melatonin inhibitory effect together with the fact that the tissue integrity seems to be necessary, suggest that in the retina, melatonin modulates NOS activity through a receptor-mediated mechanism, but not through its binding to calmodulin. The reasons of this discrepancy are not clear. It should be noted that the retina, unlike the cerebellum, the hypothalamus, or the striatum, is able to synthesize melatonin. Being a highly lipophilic molecule, melatonin has the capability of crossing all physiological barriers. However, these results suggest that the effect of melatonin on NOS activity could be restricted to those cell types that co-express melatonin receptors and NOS.

Besides NOS, another limiting step in NO synthesis is the availability of its precursor, L-arginine, which depends on the presence and activity of a specific uptake system. Physiological concentrations of melatonin significantly decrease retinal L-arginine influx (Sáenz et al., 2002). The lower Vmax of this mechanism observed in the presence of the methoxyindole suggests that melatonin decreases the number of active transporter molecules, without changing their affinity. Since melatonin decreases both L-arginine influx and its conversion to NO, a decrease in L-arginine-induced response is expectable in the presence of the methoxyindole. Indeed, the increase in cGMP accumulation induced by L-arginine is significantly reduced by melatonin (Sáenz et al., 2002). Despite the fact that NO donors, such as sodium nitroprusside releases NO in a NOS-independent way, we showed that melatonin also decreases its effect on cGMP accumulation, probably through its capacity to directly scavenge NO (Sáenz et al., 2002). In agreement with these results, it was shown that uncontrolled NO elevation causes morphological and nuclear changes in the retina and that melatonin significantly suppresses the NO induced increase in mean inner retinal layer thickness, nuclei in the inner nuclear layer, as well as the number of retinas expressing hyperchromatic expression, and apoptotic ganglion cells (Siu et al., 2004). In addition, it was demonstrated that melatonin reduces NO-induced lipid peroxidation in rat retinal homogenates (Siu et al., 1999). Peroxynitrite is a toxic oxidant formed from the reaction of superoxide and NO under conditions of inflammation and oxidant stress, and it was shown that melatonin is a scavenger of peroxynitrite (Gilad et al., 1997). Furthermore, it was demonstrated that melatonin is protective against oxidative damage in situations where NO is known to account for molecular destruction (Cuzzocrea et al., 2000).

Besides the already mentioned effects, several other mechanisms could be involved in the anti-inflammatory effect of melatonin, like inhibition of activity and expression of COX (Martínez-Campa et al., 2009), and PG release (Pawlikowski et al., 1984), inhibition of the rolling and adherence of leukocytes to endothelial layers, limiting cell migration (Markus et al., 2007), reduction of proinflammatory (Escames et al., 2006) and increase in anti-inflamatory cytokines (such as IL-1, IL-6 and IL-12), (Maestroni, 2001), decrease in vascular endothelial growth factor (Kaur et al., 2007) and chemokines levels (Park et al., 2007), and reduction of Fas ligand-mediated apoptosis, among many others, but up to now most of them were not confirmed at ocular level. Further investigations of the mechanisms by which melatonin affects its ocular targets, may unveil new concepts in ocular therapeutic.

Melatonin As a Therapeutic Resource for Uveitis Treatment

Kükner et al. (2006) and Sande et al. (2008) have investigated the effectiveness of melatonin as a therapeutic strategy in uveitis. In the Kukner study, intravitreal injections of bovine serum albumin were used to induce uveitis in the guinea pig. Melatonin, vitamin E, or aprotinin were intraperitoneally administered 3 days after albumin injection. A significant increase in leptin expression occurs in the retina, choroid, sclera, and episclera; ganglion cells were edematous and inner plexiform layer thickness increased in uveitic eyes. In animals treated with melatonin, vitamin E, or aprotinin, leptin expression was similar to the control group and edema and histopathological changes were reduced (Kükner et al., 2006). Sande et al. studied EIU, another established experimental model for uveitis, giving a single intravitreal injection of LPS in the golden hamster. In this study, a pellet of melatonin was implanted subcutaneously 2 h before the intravitreal injection of LPS. Twenty-four hours and 8 days after injection, the inflammatory response was evaluated in terms of: (i) integrity of BOB, (ii) clinical signs, (iii) histopathological studies, and (iv) retinal function. Melatonin reduced the leakage of proteins and cells in the anterior segment of LPS-injected eyes, decreased clinical signs, and protected the ultrastructure of BOBs. In animals injected with LPS, a remarkable disorganization of rod outer segment membranous disks was observed, whereas no morphological changes in photoreceptor outer segments were observed in animals treated with LPS plus melatonin. Furthermore, melatonin prevented the decrease in the ERG activity induced by LPS. Melatonin significantly abrogated the LPS-induced increase in retinal NOS activity, TNFα, and nuclear factor κB (NFκB) p50 and p65 subunits levels (Sande et al., 2008). These results indicate that melatonin prevents clinical, biochemical, histological, ultrastructural, and functional consequences of experimental uveitis in hamsters, probably through an NFκB-dependent mechanism. More recently, we studied the anti-inflammatory effect of melatonin administered after the onset of ocular inflammation in the golden hamster (Sande et al., 2014). For this purpose, hamster eyes were intravitreally injected with vehicle or LPS, and melatonin (10 mg/kg) was intraperitoneally supplied every 24 h, starting 12 h or 24 h post-LPS injection. The results indicate that both post-treatments with melatonin significantly decreased clinical symptoms, reduced the leakage of cells and proteins, and decreased PG levels in AH from eyes injected with LPS. In addition, melatonin avoided the decrease in scotopic ERG a- and b-wave amplitude, protected the retinal structure, and reduced the increase in NOS activity, lipid peroxidation, and TNFα levels induced by LPS (Sande et al., 2014). These observations support that melatonin could be potentially effective in patients with fully established uveitis, since it was capable of suppressing actively ongoing inflammatory responses. We have also examined the effect of melatonin on experimentally-induced feline uveitis. For this purpose, melatonin was orally administered every 24 h, from 24 h before until 45 days after intravitreal injections of vehicle or LPS (Del Sole et al., 2012). Eyes were evaluated by means of clinical evaluation, IOP, BOB integrity (*via* measurement of protein concentration and cell content in samples of AH), ERG, and histological examination of the retinas. The treatment with melatonin significantly decreased clinical signs and prevented the reduction in IOP induced by LPS. In LPS-injected eyes, melatonin significantly preserved the BOB integrity, as shown by a decrease in the number of infiltrating cells and protein concentration in the AH. Mean amplitudes of scotopic ERG a- and b-waves were significantly reduced in eyes injected with LPS, whereas melatonin significantly prevented the effect of LPS. At 45 days after injection, LPS induced alterations in photoreceptors and at the middle portion of the retina, whereas melatonin preserved the retinal structure. These results indicate that melatonin prevented clinical, biochemical, functional, and histological alterations induced by LPS injection in cats (Del Sole et al., 2012). Thus, melatonin might constitute a useful tool for the treatment of feline uveitis.

CONCLUSION

Uveitis, a disease with potentially blinding sequels remains a challenging field to clinical and veterinarian ophthalmologists as the disease causes significant morbidity and the use of traditional forms of treatment is restricted by limited effectiveness and considerable side effects. Several lines of evidence support the involvement of oxidative damage, increased NO and PGs production as pathogenic mechanisms of uveitis. Melatonin by itself exhibits both antioxidant and antinitridergic properties, and has the ability to reduce PG levels, among many other anti-inflammatory effects. As mentioned before, ocular inflammation is mainly treated with topical and/or systemic application of corticosteroids. During long-term treatment with corticosteroids, however, care must be taken to guard against both ocular and systemic complications such as cataract, cortisonic glaucoma, diabetes, and immunosuppressive effect. Therefore, the establishment of additive anti-inflammatory approaches is desirable to decrease the rate and degree of these complications. The results obtained in hamsters and cats strongly support that melatonin, which lacks of adverse collateral effects even at high doses, could be a promissory resource in the management of uveitis. Alone or combined with corticosteroid therapy, the anti-inflammatory effects melatonin may benefit patients with chronic uveitis and decrease the rate and degree of corticosteroid-induced complications. Although in the mentioned studies in cats (Del Sole et al., 2012) only the preventive effect of melatonin in feline experimental uveitis was demonstrated, this "relative weakness" does not preclude its clinical relevance. Indeed, uveitis is a common consequence of ocular surgery (cataract surgery and vitrectomy, among others). Thus, even as preventive strategy, the present results suggest that melatonin, a very safe compound for human and cat use, should be included in the ophthalmic therapeutic resources. Moreover, as already mentioned, a post-treatment with melatonin significantly attenuates ocular inflammation induced by LPS in golden hamsters. In summary, melatonin appears as a potentially useful anti-inflammatory drug, particularly in ophthalmology, and as an alternative or eventually as complement to glucocorticoids, since it resulted to be highly effective and it does not present the side effects of these steroids.

References

Acuña-Castroviejo, D; Escames, G; Leon, J; et al. Mitochondrial regulation by melatonin and its metabolites. *Adv Exp Med Biol.*, 2003, 527, 549-557.

Adler, LJ; Gyulai, FE; Diehl, DJ; et al. Regional brain activity changes associated with fentanyl analgesia elucidated by positron emission tomography. *Anesth Analg.*, 1997, 84, 120-126.

Barnett, KC; Crispin, SM. Tracto uveal. In: Barnett, KC; Crispin, SM; eds. Oftalmología Felina atlas & texto. Buenos Aires: Intermédica, 2000, 118-139.

Becquet, F; Courtois, Y; Goureau, O. Nitric oxide in the eye: multifaceted roles and diverse outcomes. *Surv Ophthalmol.*, 1997, 42, 71-82.

Belforte, N; Moreno, MC; Cymeryng, C; et al. Effect of ocular hypertension on retinal |nitridergic pathway activity. *Invest Ophthalmol Vis Sci.*, 2007, 48, 2127-2133.

Belforte, NA; Moreno, MC; de Zavalía, N; et al. Melatonin: a novel neuroprotectant for the treatment of glaucoma. *J Pineal Res.*, 2010, 48, 353-364.

Bellhorn, RW. Permeability of blood-ocular barriers of neonatal and adult cat to sodium fluorescein. *Invest Ophthalmol Vis Sci.*, 1980, 19, 870-877.

Bellot, JL; Palmero, M; Garcia-Cabanes, C; et al. Additive effect of nitric oxide and prostaglandin-E2 synthesis inhibitors in endotoxin-induced uveitis in the rabbit. *Inflamm Res.*, 1996, 45, 203-208.

Bettahi, I; Pozo, D; Osuna, C; et al. Melatonin reduces nitric oxide synthase activity in rat hypothalamus. *J Pineal Res.*, 1996, 20, 205-210.

Bhattacherjee P. Prostaglandins and inflammatory reactions in the eye. *Methods Find Exp Clin Pharmacol.*, 1980, 2, 17-31.

Bosch-Morell, F; Roma, J; Marin, N; et al. Role of oxygen and nitrogen species in experimental uveitis: anti-inflammatory activity of the synthetic antioxidant ebselen. *Free Radic Biol Med.*, 2002, 33, 669-675.

Breitschwerdt, EB; Abrams-Ogg, AC; Lappin, MR; Bienzle, D; Hancock, SI; Cowan, SM; Clooten, JK; Hegarty, BC; Hawkins, EC. Molecular evidence supporting Ehrlichia canis-like infection in cats. *J Vet Intern Med.*, 2002, 16, 642-649.

Cassin, B; Rubin, M. Dictionary of eye terminology. 4th edition. Gainesville (FL): Triad Publishing Company, 2001.

Cardinali, DP; Rosner, JM. Metabolism of serotonin by the rat retina in vitro. *J Neurochem.*, 1971, 18, 1769-1770.

Cardinali, DP; Rosner, JM. Retinal localization of the hydroxyindole-O-methyl transferase (HIOMT) in the rat. *Endocrinology*, 1971, 89, 301-303.

Celebi, S; Dilsiz, N; Yilmaz, T; Kukner, AS. Effects of melatonin, vitamin E and octreotide on lipid peroxidation during ischemia-reperfusion in the guinea pig retina. *Eur J Ophthalmol.*, 2002, 12, 77-83.

Chavkin, M; Lappin, M; Powell, C; et al. Seroepidemiologic and clinical observations of 93 cases of uveitis in cats. *Prog Vet Comp Ophthalmol.*, 1992, 2, 29-36.

Chi, ZL; Hayasaka, S; Zhang, XY; et al. Effects of rolipram, a selective inhibitor of type 4 phosphodiesterase, on lipopolysaccharide-induced uveitis in rats. *Invest Ophthalmol Vis Sci.*, 2004, 45, 2497-2502.

Colitz, CMH. Feline Uveitis: Diagnosis and Treatment. *Clin Tech Small Anim Pract*, 2005, 20, 117-120.

Collins, BK; Moore, CP (1999). Disease and surgery of the canine anterior uvea, pp 151-81. *En*: K.N. Gelatt (ed.) Veterinary Ophthalmology, Tercera Edición. Lippincott Williams Wilkins. Philadelphia.

Csukas, S; Paterson, CA; Brown, K; et al. Time course of rabbit ocular inflammatory response and mediator release after intravitreal endotoxin. *Invest Ophthalmol Vis Sci.*, 1990, 31, 382-387.

Curtis, R; Barnett, K; Lewis, S. Clinical and pathological observations concerning the aetiology of primary lens luxation in the dog. *Vet Rec.*, 1983, 112, 238-246.

Cuzzocrea, S; Costantino, G; Gitto, E; et al. Protective effects of melatonin in ischemic brain injury. *J Pineal Res.*, 2000, 29, 217-227.

Davidson, MG; Lappin, MR; English, RV; et al. A feline model of ocular toxoplasmosis. *Invest Ophthalmol Vis Sci.*, 1993, 34, 3653-3660.

de Vos, AF; Klaren, VN; Kijlstra, A. Expression of multiple cytokines and IL-1RA in the uvea and retina during endotoxin-induced uveitis in the rat. *Invest Ophthalmol Vis Sci.*, 1994, 35, 3873-3883.

Davidson, MG; Nasisse, MP; English, RV; Wilcock, BP; Jamieson, VE. Feline anterior uveitis: A study of 53 cases. *J Am Anim Hosp Assoc.*, 1991, 22, 77–83.

Del Sole, MJ; Sande, PH; Bernades, JM; Aba, MA; Rosenstein, RE. Circadian rhythm of intraocular pressure in cats. *Vet Ophthalmol.*, 2007, 10, 155-61.

Del Sole, MJ; Sande, PH; Felipe, AE; Fernandez, DC; et al. Characterization of uveitis induced by use of a single intravitreal injection of bacterial lipopolysaccharide in cats. *Am J Vet Res.*, 2008, 11, 1487-1495.

Del Sole, MJ; Sande, JM; Fernandez, DC; et al. Therapeutic benefit of melatonin in experimental feline uveitis. *J Pineal Res.*, 2012, 52, 29-37.

Dubocovich, ML. Melatonin is a potent modulator of dopamine release in the retina. *Nature*, 1983, 306, 782-784.

Eagle, R; Spencer, W. Lens. In: Spencer, W; editor. Ophthalmic pathology. 4th edition. Philadelphia: WB Saunders; 1996. p. 372-427.

Escames, G; Acuña-Castroviejo, D; López, LC; et al. Pharmacological utility of melatonin in the treatment of septic shock: experimental and clinical evidence. *J Pharm Pharmacol.*, 2006, 58, 1153-1165.

Faillace, MP; Sarmiento, MI; Siri, LN; Rosenstein, RE. Diurnal variations in cyclic AMP and melatonin content of golden hamster retina. *J Neurochem.*, 1994, 62, 1995-2000.

Faillace, MP; Cutrera, R; Sarmiento, MI; Rosenstein, RE. Evidence for local synthesis of melatonin in golden hamster retina. *Neuroreport.*, 1995, 6, 2093-2095.

Flach, A. Cyclo-oxygenase inhibitors in ophthalmology. *Surv Ophthalmol.*, 1992, 36, 259-284.

Forrester, JV; Worgul, BV; Merriam, GR; Jr. Endotoxin-induced uveitis in the rat. *Albrecht Von Graefes Arch Klin Ophthalmol.*, 1980, 213, 221-233.

Gelatt, K; Boggess, T; Cure, T. Evaluation of mydriatics in the cat. *J Am Anim Hosp Assoc.*, 1973, 9, 283-287.

Gemensky, A; Lorimer, D; Blanchard, G. Feline uveitis: a retrospective study of 45 cases. Presented at Annual Meeting of the American College of Veterinary Ophthalmologists 1996.

Gilad, E; Cuzzocrea, S; Zingarelli, B; Salzman, AL; Szabó, C. Melatonin is a scavenger of peroxynitrite. *Life Sci.*, 1997, 60, 169-174.

Giuliano, E. Nonsteroidal anti-inflammatory drugs in veterinary ophthalmology. *Vet Clin North Am Small Anim Pract.*, 2004, 34, 707-723.

Glaze, MB; Gelatt, KN. Feline ophthalmology. In: Gelatt, KN; ed. Veterinary ophthalmology. 3th ed. Philadelphia: Lippincott Williams & Wilkins, 1998, 1018-1025.

Goto, H; Wu, GS; Gritz, DC; et al. Chemotactic activity of the peroxidized retinal membrane lipids in experimental autoimmune uveitis. *Curr Eye Res.*, 1991, 10, 1009-1014.

Goureau, O; Bellot, J; Thillaye, B; et al. Increased nitric oxide production in endotoxin-induced uveitis: reduction of uveitis by an inhibitor of nitric oxide synthase. *J Immunol.*, 1995, 154, 6518-6523.

Guajardo, MH; Terrasa, AM; Catala, A. Protective effect of indoleamines on in vitro ascorbate-Fe2+ dependent lipid peroxidation of rod outer segment membranes of bovine retina. *J Pineal Res.*, 2003, 35, 276-282.

Guenther, AL; Schmidt, SI; Laatsch, H; et al. Reactions of the melatonin metabolite AMK (N1-acetyl-5-methoxykynuramine) with reactive nitrogen species: formation of novel compounds, 3-acetamidomethyl-6-methoxycinnolinone and 3-nitro-AMK. *J Pineal Res.*, 2005, 39, 251-260.

Gum, GG; Gelatt, KN; Esson, DW. Physiology of the Eye. In: Gelatt, KN; ed. *Veterinary ophthalmology*. 4th ed. Blackwell Publishing, Iowa, 2007, 149-182.

Gunn-Moore, DA; Jenkins, PA; Lucke, VM. Feline tuberculosis: a literature review and discussion of 19 cases caused by an unusual mycobacterial variant. *Vet Res.*, 1996, 138, 53-58.

Hamasaki, DI; Sato, H; Santhanakrishnan, S; Shinohara, T. Correlation between the physiologic and morphologic changes in experimental autoimmune uveitis induced by peptide G of S antigen. *Invest Ophthalmol Vis Sci.*, 1993, 34, 1861-1871.

Hardeland, R; Balzer, I; Poeggeler, B; et al. On the primary functions of melatonin in evolution: mediation of photoperiodic signals in a unicell, photooxidation, and scavenging of free radicals. *J Pineal Res.*, 1995, 18, 104-111.

Hardeland, R. Antioxidative protection by melatonin: multiplicity of mechanisms from radical detoxification to radical avoidance. *Endocrine*, 2005, 27, 119-130.

Harris, BP; Miller, PE; Bloss, JR; Pellittieri, PJ. Ophthalmomyasis interna anterior associated with *Cuterebra* spp in a cat. *J Am Vet Med Assoc.*, 2000, 216, 352-355.

Hashida, M; Fukushima, A; Zhang, J; et al. Involvement of superoxide generated by polymorphonuclear leukocytes in endotoxin-induced uveitis. *Graefes Arch Clin Exp Ophthalmol.*, 2000, 238, 359-365.

Hoekzema, R; Murray, PI; van Haren, MA; et al. Analysis of interleukin-6 in endotoxin-induced uveitis. *Invest Ophthalmol Vis Sci.*, 1991, 32, 88-95.

Holmberg, B; Maggs, D. The use of corticosteroids to treat ocular inflammation. *Vet Clin North Am Small Anim Pract.*, 2004, 34, 693-705.

Horio, N; Terasaki, H; Yamamoto, E; Miyake, Y. Electroretinogram in the diagnosis of endophthalmitis after intraocular lens implantation. *Am J Ophthalmol.*, 2001, 132, 258-259.

Howes, EL; Jr; McKay, DG. The effects of aspirin and indomethacin on the ocular response to circulating bacterial endotoxin in the rabbit. *Invest Ophthalmol.*, 1976, 15, 648-651.

Ianas, O; Olinescu, R; Badescu, I. Melatonin involvement in oxidative processes. *Endocrinologie*, 1991, 29, 147-153.

Jacquemin, E ; De Kozak, Y ; Thillaye, B ; et al. Expression of inducible nitric oxide synthase in the eye from endotoxin-induced uveitis rats. *Invest Ophthalmol Vis Sci.*, 1996, 37, 1187-1196.

Johnson, BW; Helper, LC; Szajerski, ME. Intraocular *Cuterebra* in a cat. *J Am Vet Med Assoc.*, 1988, 193, 829-830.

Kashiwagi, K; Iizuka, Y; Tanaka, Y; et al. Dual action of nitric oxide on purely isolated retinal ganglion cells. *Curr Eye Res.*, 2001, 23, 233-239

Kaur, C; Sivakumar, V; Yong, Z; et al. Blood-retinal barrier disruption and ultrastructural changes in the hypoxic retina in adult rats: the beneficial effect of melatonin administration. *J Pathol.*, 2007, 212, 429-439.

Kim, IT; Park, SK; Lim, JH. Inflammatory response in experimental Staphylococcus and *Pseudomonas* endophthalmitis. *Ophthalmologica*, 1999, 213, 305-310.

Klauss, G; Constantinescu, G. Nonhypotensive autonomic agents in veterinary ophthalmology. *Vet Clin North Am Small Anim Pract.*, 2004, 34, 777-800.

Kogiso, M; Tanouchi, Y; Mimura, Y; et al. Endotoxin-induced uveitis in mice. 1. Induction of uveitis and role of T lymphocytes. *Jpn J Ophthalmol.,* 1992, 36, 281-290.

Kükner, A; Colakoğlu, N; Serin, D; et al. Effects of intraperitoneal vitamin E, melatonin and aprotinin on leptin expression in the guinea pig eye during experimental uveitis. *Acta Ophthalmol Scand.*, 2006, 84, 54-61.

Kurihara, T; Ozawa, Y; Shinoda, K; et al. Neuroprotective effects of angiotensin II type 1 receptor (AT1R) blocker, telmisartan, via modulating AT1R and AT2R signaling in retinal inflammation. *Invest Ophthalmol Vis Sci.*, 2006, 47, 5545-5552.

Lappin, MR; Marks, A; Greene, CE; et al. Serologic prevalence of selected infectious diseases in cats with uveitis. *J Am Vet Med Assoc.*, 1992, 201, 1005-1009.

Lappin, MR; Black, JC. Bartonella spp infection as a possible cause of uveitis in a cat. *J Am Vet Med Assoc.*, 1999, 214, 1205–7, 1200.

Lappin, MR. Feline infectious uveitis. *J Feline Med Surg.*, 2000, 2, 159-163.

Lee, MC; Chung, YT; Lee, JH; et al. Antioxidant effect of melatonin in human retinal neuron cultures. *Exp Neurol.*, 2001, 172, 407-415.

Leiva, M; Lloret, A; Peña, T; Roura, X. Therapy of ocular and visceral leishmaniasis in a cat. *Vet Ophthalmol.*, 2005, 8, 71-75.

León, J; Vives, F; Crespo, E; Camacho, E; Espinosa, A; Gallo, MA; Escames, G; Acuña-Castroviejo, D. Modification of nitric oxide synthase activity and neuronal response in rat striatum by melatonin and kynurenine derivatives. *J Neuroendocrinol.*, 1998, 10, 297-302.

León, J; Acuña-Castroviejo, D; Escames, G; et al. Melatonin mitigates mitochondrial malfunction. *J Pineal Res.*, 2005, 38, 1-9.

León, J; Acuña-Castroviejo, D; Sainz, RM; et al. Melatonin and mitochondrial function. *Life Sci.*, 2004, 75, 765-790.

Leonardi, A; Busato, F; Fregona, I; et al. Anti-inflammatory and antiallergic effects of ketorolac tromethamine in the conjunctival provocation model. *Br J Ophthalmol.*, 2000, 84, 1228-1232.

Liang, FQ; Green, L; Wang, C; et al. Melatonin protects human retinal pigment epithelial (RPE) cells against oxidative stress. *Exp Eye Res.*, 2004, 78, 1069-1075.

Maggs, D. Feline uveitis: An "intraocular lymphadenopathy". *Journal of Feline Medicine and Surgery*, 2009, 11, 167-182.

Magnarelli, LA; Bushmich, SL; Ijdo, JW; Fikrig, E. Seroprevalence of antibodies against Borrelia burgdorferi and Anaplasma phagocytophilum in cats. *Am J Vet Res.*, 2005, 66, 1895-1899.

Mandai, M; Yoshimura, N; Yoshida, M; et al. The role of nitric oxide synthase in endotoxin-induced uveitis: effect of N^G-nitro L-arginine. *Invest Ophthalmol Vis Sci.*, 1994, 35, 3673-3681.

Marchiafava, PL; Longoni, B. Melatonin as an antioxidant in retinal photoreceptors. *J Pineal Res.*, 1999, 26, 184-189.

Markus, RP; Ferreira, ZS; Fernandes, PA; Cecon, E. The immune-pineal axis: a shuttle between endocrine and paracrine melatonin sources. *Neuroimmunomodulation.*, 2007, 14, 126-133.

Martin, XD; Malina, HZ; Brennan, MC; Hendrickson, PH; Lichter, PR. The ciliary body--the third organ found to synthesize indoleamines in humans. *Eur J Ophthalmol.*, 1992, 2, 67-72

Martínez-Campa, C; González, A; Mediavilla, MD; et al. Melatonin inhibits aromatase promoter expression by regulating cyclooxygenases expression and activity in breast cancer cells. *Br J Cancer*, 2009, 101, 1613-1619.

Masferrer, JL; Kulkarni, PS. Cyclooxygenase-2 inhibitors: a new approach to the therapy of ocular inflammation. *Surv Ophthalmol.*, 1997, 41, 35-40.

Mhatre, MC1; van Jaarsveld, AS; Reiter, RJ. Melatonin in the lacrimal gland: first demonstration and experimental manipulation. *Biochem Biophys Res Commun.*, 1988, 30, 153, 1186-1192.

Millichamp, N; Dziezyc, J; Rhohde, B; et al. Acute effects of anti-inflammatory drugs on neodymium:nyttrium aluminum garnet laser-induced uveitis in dogs. *Am J Vet Res.*, 1991, 52, 1279-1284.

Olivero, DK; Riis, RD; Dutton, AG; et al. Feline lens displacement: a retrospective analysis of 345 cases. *Prog Vet Comp Ophthalmol*, 1991, 1, 239-244.

Pandi-Perumal, SR; Srinivasan, V; Maestroni, GJ; et al. Melatonin: Nature's most versatile biological signal? *FEBS J.*, 2006, 273, 2813-2838.

Paredes, SD; Bejarano, I; Terrón, MP; Barriga, C; Reiter, RJ; Rodríguez, AB. Melatonin and tryptophan counteract lipid peroxidation and modulate superoxide dismutase activity in ringdove heterophils in vivo. Effect of antigen-induced activation and age. Age (Dordr)., 2009, 31, 179-188.

Park, HJ; Kim, HJ; Ra, J; et al. Melatonin inhibits lipopolysaccharide-induced chemokine subfamily gene expression in human peripheral blood mononuclear cells in a microarray analysis. *J Pineal Res.*, 2007, 43, 121-129.

Parks, DJ; Cheung, MK; Chan, CC; Roberge, FG. The role of nitric oxide in uveitis. *Arch Ophthalmol.*, 1994, 112, 544-546.

Pawlikowski, M; Juszczak, M; Karasek, E; et al. Melatonin inhibits prostaglandin E release from the medial basal hypothalamus of pinealectomized rats. *J Pineal Res.*, 1984, 1, 317-321.

Peiffer, RL; Wilcock, BP. Histopathologic study of uveitis in cats: 139 cases (1978-1988). *J Am Vet Med Assoc.*, 1991, 198, 135-138.

Perianin, A; Roch-Arveiller, M; Giround, J; et al. In vivo effects of indomethacin and flurbiprofen on the locomotion of neutrophils elicited by immune and non-immune inflammation in the rat. *Eur J Pharmacol.*, 1985, 106, 327-333.

Pierce, ME; Besharse, JC. Circadian regulation of retinomotor movements. I. Interaction of melatonin and dopamine in the control of cone length. *J Gen Physiol.*, 1985, 86, 671-689.

Planck, SR; Huang, XN; Robertson, JE; Rosenbaum, JT. Cytokine mRNA levels in rat ocular tissues after systemic endotoxin treatment. *Invest Ophthalmol Vis Sci.*, 1994, 35, 924-930.

Poeggeler, B; Reiter, RJ; Tan, DX; et al. Melatonin, hydroxyl radical-mediated oxidative damage, and aging: a hypothesis. *J Pineal Res.*, 1993, 14,
151-168.

Powell, CC; Lappin, MR. Diagnosis and treatment of feline uveitis. *Comp Cont Educ Pract.*, 2001, 23, 258-266.

Pozo, D; Reiter, RJ; Calvo, JC; et al. Inhibition of cerebellar nitric oxide synhtase and cyclic GMP production by melatonin via complex formation with calmodulin. *J Cell Biochem.*, 1997, 65, 430-442.

Rao, NA; Patchett, R; Fernandez, MA; et al. Treatment of experimental granulomatous uveitis by lipoxygenase and cyclo-oxygenase inhibitors. *Arch Ophthalmol.*, 1987, 105, 413-415.

Rao, NA. Role of oxygen free radicals in retinal damage associated with experimental uveitis. *Trans Am Ophthalmol Soc.*, 1990, 88, 797-850.

Reiter, RJ; Garcia, JJ; Pie, J. Oxidative toxicity in models of neurodegeneration: responses to melatonin. *Restor Neurol Neurosci.*, 1998, 12, 135-142.

Reiter, RJ; Guerrero, JM; Escames, G; et al. Prophylactic actions of melatonin in oxidative neurotoxicity. *Ann NY Acad Sci.*, 1997, 825, 70-78.

Reiter, RJ; Tan, DX; Mayo, JC; et al. Melatonin as an antioxidant: biochemical mechanisms and pathophysiological implications in humans. *Acta Biochim Pol.*, 2003, 50, 1129-1146.

Reiter, RJ; Tan, DX; Osuna, C; Gitto, E. Actions of melatonin in the reduction of oxidative stress. A review. *J Biomed Sci.*, 2000, 7, 444-458.

Reiter, RJ; Tan, DX; Poeggeler, B; et al. Melatonin as a free radical scavenger: implications for aging and age-related diseases. *Ann NY Acad Sci.*, 1994, 719, 1-12.

Richter, Schaarschmidt-Kiener, Krudewig. Ocular signs, diagnosis and long-term treatment with allopurinol in a cat with leishmaniasis. *Schweiz Arch Tierheilkd.*, 2014, 156, 289-294.

Rosenbaum, JT; McDevitt, HO; Guss, RB; et al. Endotoxin-induced uveitis in rats as a model for human disease. *Nature,* 1980, 286, 611-613.

Rufiange, M; Dumont, M; Lachapelle, P. Correlating retinal function with melatonin secretion in subjects with an early or late circadian phase. *Invest Ophthalmol Vis Sci.*, 2002, 43, 2491-2499.

Sáenz, DA; Goldin, AP; Minces, L; et al. Effect of melatonin on the retinal glutamate/glutamine cycle in the golden hamster retina. *FASEB J.*, 2004, 18, 1912-1913.

Sáenz, DA; Turjanski, AG; Sacca, GB; et al. Physiological concentrations of melatonin inhibit the nitridergic pathway in the Syrian hamster retina. *J Pineal Res.*, 2002, 33, 31-36.

Sande, PH; Fernandez, DC; Aldana Marcos, HJ; et al. Therapeutic effect of melatonin in experimental uveitis. *Am J Pathol.*, 2008, 173, 1702-1713.

Sande, PH1; Dorfman, D; Fernandez, DC; Chianelli, M; Domínguez Rubio, AP; Franchi, AM; Silberman, DM; Rosenstein RE, Sáenz DA. The post-treatment with melatonin attenuates experimental ocular inflammation. *Br J Pharmacol.* 2014. doi: 10.1111/bph.12873.

Saraswathy, S; Rao, NA. Photoreceptor mitochondrial oxidative stress in experimental autoimmune uveitis. *Ophthalmic Res.*, 2008, 40, 160-164.

Satici, A; Guzey, M; Gurler, B; et al. Malondialdehyde and antioxidant enzyme levels in the aqueous humor of rabbits in endotoxin-induced uveitis. *Eur J Ophthalmol.*, 2003, 13, 779-783.

Scher, J; Wankiewicz, E; Brown, GM; Fujieda, H. MT(1) melatonin receptor in the human retina: expression and localization. *Invest. Ophthalmol Vis Sci.*, 2002, 43, 889-897.

Sennlaub, F; Courtois, Y; Goureau, O. Inducible nitric oxide synthase mediates retinal apoptosis in ischemic proliferative retinopathy. *J Neurosci.*, 2002, 22, 3987-3993.

Siu, AW; Ortiz, GG; Benitez-King, G; et al. Effects of melatonin on the nitric oxide treated retina. *Br J Ophthalmol.*, 2004, 88, 1078-1081.

Siu, AW; Reiter, RJ; To, CH. Pineal indoleamines and vitamin E reduce nitric oxide-induced lipid peroxidation in rat retinal homogenates *J Pineal Res.*, 1999, 2, 122-128.

Stiles, J; Townsend, WM. Feline ophthalmology. In: Gelatt KN, editor. 4th edition, Veterinary ophthalmology, vol. 2. Ames (IA): Blackwell Publishing; 2007. p. 1117-1124.

Stevenson, L; Matesanz, N; Colhoun, L; et al. Reduced nitro-oxidative stress and neural cell death suggests a protective role for microglial cells in TNFalpha-/- mice in ischemic retinopathy. *Invest. Ophthalmol Vis Sci.*, 2010, 51, 3291-3299.

Streeten, B. Pathology of the lens. In: Albert D, Jakobiec F, editors. Principles and practice of ophthalmology. Philadelphia: WB Saunders; 2000. p. 3685-749.

Tan, DX; Manchester, LC; Terron, MP; et al. One molecule, many derivatives: a never-ending interaction of melatonin with reactive oxygen and nitrogen species? *J Pineal Res.*, 2007, 42, 28-42.

Tosini, G; Menaker, M. The clock in the mouse retina: melatonin synthesis and photoreceptor degeneration. *Brain Res.*, 1998, 789, 221-228.

Turjanski, AG; Chaia, Z; Doctorovich, F; et al. N-Nitrosomelatonin. *Acta Crystallogr C.*, 2000, 56, 682-683.

Turjanski, AG; Leonik, F; Estrin, DA; et al. Scavenging of NO by Melatonin. *J Am Chem Soc.*, 2000, 122, 10468-10469.

Verneuil, M. Ocular leishmaniasis in a cat: case report. *J Fr Ophtalmol.*, 2013, 36, e67-72.

Ward, D; Ferguson, D; Ward, S; et al. Comparison of the blood-aqueous barrier stabilizing effects of steroidal and nonsteroidal anti-inflammatory agents in the dog. *Prog Vet Comp Ophthalmol*, 1992, 2, 117-124.

Ward, D. Comparative efficacy of topically applied flurbiprofen, diclofenac, tolmetin, and suprofen for the treatment of experimentally induced blood-aqueous barrier disruption in dogs. *Am J Vet Res.*, 1996, 57, 875-878.

Wilkie, DA. Control of ocular inflammation. *Vet Clin North Am Small Anim Pract.*, 1990, 20, 693-713.

Wilkie, DA. Trastornos de la úvea. In: Kirk RW, Bonagura JD, eds. Terapéutica veterinaria de pequeños animales XI. Madrid: McGraw-Hill Interamericana, 1994, 1233-1240.

Wu, GS; Sevanian, A; Rao, NA. Detection of retinal lipid hydroperoxides in experimental uveitis. *Free Radic Biol Med.*, 1992, 12, 1927.

Yomura, Y; Shoji, Y; Asai, D; et al. Direct, real-time, simultaneous monitoring of intravitreal nitric oxide and oxygen in endotoxininduced uveitis in rabbits. *Life Sci.*, 2007, 80, 1449-1457.

Zhan, GL; Miranda, OC; Bito, LZ. Steroid glaucoma: corticosteroid-induced ocular hypertension in cats. *Exp Eye Res.*, 1992, 54, 211-218.

INDEX

B

C

D

G

H

I

J

K

L

O

P

Q

R

S

T

U

V

W